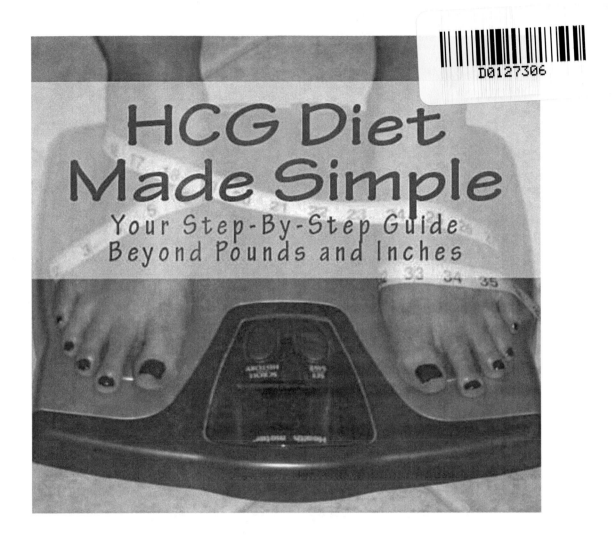

HCG Diet Made Simple

Your Step-By-Step Guide Beyond Pounds and Inches

By

Harmony Clearwater Grace

Dear hCG Diet Friends,

After reading *The Weight Loss Cure* by Kevin Trudeau, I was sold on the concepts that he presented, but had no idea how to actually put the plan into action. After much research, I have uncovered many resources not mentioned in the book that have helped me to start my weight reduction adventure with hCG. I've already reduced 50 pounds, after being unsuccessful with every other diet that I have tried over the last 9 years. Using this weight reduction method, I expect to lose the entire 100 extra pounds that I've been carrying around. FINALLY, a CURE for the problem that has plagued me for almost a decade now!

You see, most of my life, I weighed in at 120 pounds. Even for my 5'6" small-boned frame, that was considered underweight, although it was my normal weight that my body maintained without effort. I could eat anything I wanted, as much as I wanted, and I never gained weight. My boyfriends would pester me to gain some weight, but I was already eating everything in sight with no gain. One of them pestered me so much about it that I got so nervous that I LOST weight.

Enter Depo-Provera. I took this birth control shot ONCE at the age of 38. I immediately began gaining weight after the shot. I panicked and began modifying my eating habits, but I had no idea how to lose weight, because I'd never had to do it in all my 38 years. I tried all kinds of diets, but no matter what I did, I continued to gain. My menstrual periods didn't come back for 14 months, which to me indicated that my hormones were tilted off-kilter in a big way. I talked to my friends about it, learning that the daughter of one of my friends had also taken the shot and gained 20 pounds in a month. She was another one of those "never gain, eat like a horse" type of girls that everyone envied. I started to suspect that I was in deep trouble now.

I found a book by the title of *Birth Control By Injection: The Story of Depo-Provera*, in which I read the words "knockout blow to the pituitary" used with reference to Depo-Provera in Chapter Five. The book was written by an endocrinologist named T. J. Vecchio, M.D., F.A.C.P., who organized international clinical trials with Depo-Provera over a 10 year period, as well as conducting such trials on his own. He wrote a number of scientific articles on the subject, including the lead article on "Long-Acting Injectable Contraceptives" for the 1976 issue of *Advances in Steroid Biochemistry and*

Pharmacology, as well as making numerous oral presentations on the subject to medical groups around the world.

Now, I was really concerned, and with good cause, as it turned out. That same chapter outlined the effects of Depo-Provera on the adrenal glands. Within six years, I had been diagnosed with Chronic Fatigue Syndrome and had gained 100 pounds. My medical doctor could not give me any hope or effective treatment. The naturopathic doctor that I turned to next explained that he had been treating CFS/CFIDS for over 50 years and had originally called it Adrenal Syndrome because it was caused by over-stimulation of the HPA (hypothalamus/pituitary/adrenal) axis by chronic stress or a genetic predisposition to weak adrenals. I knew that my adrenals had been weakened by the Depo-Provera along with the rest of my endocrine system. My metabolism had been ruined as well, causing the weight to pack on, no matter what I tried in my efforts to stop it. The methods that I used for my CFS/CFIDS recovery did absolutely nothing to help me with weight reduction, however. The solution for my CFS/CFIDS is the subject of another book that I will write soon, but in this book I want to concentrate on the solution to my weight issues.

I've included links to such helpful references as Dr. A. T. W. Simeons' original manuscript from which Kevin learned about the cure. Also, you will find recipes to use during the injection phase to help make it less repetitive, as well as sources for an oral (sublingual) version of hCG if the mere thought of injections is enough to scare you away from considering using this method. This is your one-stop comprehensive companion source for practical ways to actually put the hCG diet to use for your **very own personal** weight reduction cure!

Blessings with Love,
Harmony

P.S. Also, please email me when you have reduced below 200 pounds, if you start out above that, so that I can personally tell you, "Welcome to ONE-derland! Onward and downward!! (on the scale, that is)." Any other major milestone emails are also happily welcomed!

Update: I will start back on Phase 2 soon to lose the 50 remaining pounds using hCG! For the first time in 9 years, I have not only the hope, but the assurance in my heart, that I can lose the excess weight that has been the bane of my existence for so long.

Table of Contents

Limit of Liability / Disclaimer of Warranty: While the publisher and author have used their best efforts in preparing this book, they make no representations or warranties with respect to the accuracy or completeness of the contents of this book and specifically disclaim any implied warranties or merchantability or fitness for a particular purpose. No warranty may be created or extended by sales representatives or written sales materials. The advice and strategies contained herein may not be suitable for your situation. Neither the publisher nor the author is engaged in rendering professional services, and you should consult a professional where appropriate. Neither the publisher nor the author shall be liable for any loss of profit or other commercial damages, including but not limited to special, incidental, consequential, or other damages.

Additional Disclaimers

Use this book at your own risk.

In the event that you use the information in this book without your doctor's or health practitioner's approval, you prescribe for yourself. It is my understanding that this remains your constitutional and God-given right, but I assume no responsibility for how you make use of the data in this book. I do not diagnose or prescribe. For your own safety, tell your health professional absolutely EVERYTHING that you take, even over the counter medications, to avoid any harmful interactions. Internet advice or advice from a book is not a substitute for the advice of a medical professional. Always consult your physician before beginning an exercise or diet program.

www.hcgdietmadesimple.com and/or Harmony Clearwater Grace and/or Harmonious Clarity Group, LLC cannot be held liable for any misuse of its products or recommendations. The information and images in this book are for entertainment and educational purposes. None of the listed information is to be used as advice for any medical procedure. By reading, accepting, and continuing to view this book, you acknowledge that this information is to be used for entertainment and/or educational purposes only and does not represent nor replace the advice of a doctor.

The statements in this book have not been evaluated by the Food and Drug Administration. None of the products listed or mentioned should be used as a substitute for medical advice, or to diagnose, treat or cure any illness. Always consult your personal physician before consuming any new supplements and never change any medications without his/her expressed permission. If a product or treatment is recommended in these pages, it is not intended to diagnose, treat, cure, or prevent any disease. The information contained herein is meant to be used to educate and/or entertain the reader and is in no way intended to provide individual medical advice, which must be obtained by a qualified health practitioner. All information contained in this book is received from sources believed to be accurate, but no guarantee, express or implied, can be made. Readers are encouraged to verify for themselves, and to their own satisfaction, the accuracy of all information, recommendations, conclusions, comments, opinions, or anything else contained within these pages before making any kind of decisions based upon what they have read herein. Prices, policies, procedures, and any other information given in reviews of suppliers or clinics were accurate at the time of review.

PLEASE NOTE: The law requires this statement be posted: The FDA has not approved hCG for weight loss and there is no substantial evidence that hCG is effective in the treatment of obesity.

I do, of course, respectfully disagree with the FDA.

Acknowledgements

I want to thank all of the members of my hCG Dieters support group, without whom I very much doubt that this book would have been written, many of whom have very kindly allowed me to use their experiences to enhance this book, especially David Yancey and Shalom Shick.

If you have any questions or concerns about the data in this book, I am always available through email to offer whatever help and support that I can. I am also very interested in hearing your story and how this information has helped you. Please be aware, however, that I am not a medical professional and that I cannot answer medical questions.

Please email your comments, questions that are not answered in this book, and stories of your successful weight reduction to: **hcgdietmadesimple@gmail.com**.

Abbreviations used in this book

Dr. S = A.T.W. Simeons, M.D.
Dr. B = Daniel Oscar Belluscio, M.D.
KT = Kevin Trudeau
VLCD = Very Low Calorie Diet
LCD = Low Calorie Diet
LIW = Last Injection Weight
LSDW = Last Sublingual Dose Weight
SC = Subcutaneous
SQ = Subcutaneous
IM = Intramuscular
SL = Sublingual (under the tongue)
IU = International Units, a measure of potency
cc = cubic centimeters (equal to 1 ml), a measure of volume
ml = milliliters (equal to 1 cc), a measure of volume

Testimonials to This Diet

"Nearly three years ago, I gained 80 lbs during a very stressful time. In only about 6 months, I packed on all of the weight. I was under a lot of stress and was nauseated and vomited frequently, yet I still gained the weight. For the last 3 years, I have been on a number of diets, Atkins, Weight Watchers, Bob Greene, Ultra Metabolism, Dr. Mercola's diet, Jenny Craig. I also have been doing 1 hour of kick boxing several times week (Billy Blanks, Turbo Jam, PO90) along with walking 5 miles several times a week. I also have used HydroxyCut, Accelis, Hoodia, and so many others I can't remember.

I am a respiratory therapist and walk around doing treatments for 12-hr shifts. I am only 5'3" and weighed 210 lbs and was a tight size 18. I did each diet for at least 1 month or longer with little or no weight loss. As you can see, I am a very active person. People that I worked out with were losing weight. I, on the other hand, continued to have a 48-inch waist. After 3 years of struggling, the disappointments and heartbreak of diet after diet, I had finally given up. I was so depressed. Try to imagine working so hard at something for 3 years and enduring failure after failure.

Well, today September 25, I weigh 174 and I am size 12. I lost 11 inches off my waist since June 6. I have people around me doing this protocol now, just because my scrubs are baggy. It wasn't any scientific paper that convinced them to do it. It was seeing the amazing transformation that I went through and continue to go through that convinced them that hCG does work. I have done low cal diets in the past and never lost weight that was so visible and dramatic. I usually lost the hair on my head, my skin became pasty and sallow and I had dark circles under my eyes and had hanging skin and lost all my muscle mass, I felt terrible. Not this time! My hair is thick, shiny, my nails are growing like crazy, I have energy and feel great. I still have muscle, skin is tight."

And one more testimonial to the diet:
"Since I've been aware of this HCG Protocol and have almost completed it, I see the miracles that it works with your weight and performing a metabolic recovery, I find myself getting really agitated/annoyed when someone tries to tell me and others that diet and exercise is the only way to lose weight and keep it off. There have been countless times when people have asked me about a method to lose weight that's the most effective. Of course I would recommend the HCG Protocol, I would NEVER, and I mean NEVER tell a person to do diet and exercise as a weight loss method.

Then you have others that'll intervene and tell me that the Dr. Simeons protocol is a joke and that it's really unhealthy to lose weight this way, especially a lb. a day. People who've never heard of it until I mentioned it, by the way. You break down the whole process to them of how and why the weight is lost so fast and the benefits that come from the treatment AFTERWARDS when it comes to keeping it off. They still have nothing but negative things to say. It just trips me out how people think that diet and exercise is the only way to lose weight and keep it off. It's a torturous and VERY depriving lifestyle when you try to keep weight off from dieting. I've done it so I know.

Let's not mention the things that this protocol does that diet and exercise doesn't even touch. Losing problem area fats, low hunger, fast results, resetting of the hypothalamus gland, raising your metabolism sky high, etc. I'm almost finished with this protocol and (4 days left until Phase 4), and I've never seen anything like this on any weight loss method I've used in the past. No counting calories, no superhuman willpower to keep from eating, low hunger, constant results, etc.

My thing is...if diet and exercise is the only way to lose weight and the real 'solution,' then why does the obesity rate continue to rise annually? Even though there's more people on diets and buying more exercise equipment more and more each year. Let's be real. I get frustrated, annoyed and agitated when people act like this is the solution and don't want to hear of anything else, even though it has never worked for them. I've heard countless stories from people about how they work 5 hours a day in the gym, eating rabbit food and they still don't lose weight. And others have the same story, except for they do, in fact, lose weight but gain it right back afterwards faster than they lost it, plus more. Not to mention how slow they lost it. Which is frustrating.

For anyone that's curious about this method of weight loss. THIS IS THE SOLUTION! You'll never need another diet in your life once you finish this! Exercise is always good for your body, whether you're trying to lose weight or not. It's always recommended for good overall health but it's not a weight loss solution.

Let me end by saying this. For the people that doubt this protocol, stay fat for the rest of your lives and miserable from yo-yo dieting and depriving yourselves to keep the weight off. Keep losing weight and gaining it right back. But for those that are tired of dieting and exercising only to find disappointment, and are smart enough go through this protocol...we'll enjoy living normal lives as slim people that can fully enjoy the foods that we love without constantly thinking about our weight. Now you choose..."

– Dashaun

Everything that you wanted to know, but the Weight Loss Cure book by Trudeau didn't tell you....

I want to provide a valuable resource for those who, like me, wanted to do the hCG Diet, but had no clue as to the practical aspects of how to accomplish that. I am forever grateful to Kevin Trudeau for writing his book so that I could have a way to find out about Dr. Simeons' solution to my weight problem. However, his book didn't answer many questions that I had about how to actually get started and accomplish the same results as he was able to achieve. I needed someone to walk me through how to do the diet protocol and to answer questions. It took me a great deal of time to compile all the information in this book, to give you the ultimate step by step resource that I had wished for initially.

As a moderator of an hCG Diet support group with over 12,000 members, I've noticed several questions that come up again and again. I have collected these questions with answers that are accurate based on my research. I've included the questions and answers in the appropriate Phase or Step whenever possible. I cite references whenever possible to support these answers, sometimes from the Pounds and Inches manuscript itself and sometimes from the internet. When I cite references from the internet, whenever possible I include a shortened URL using TinyURLs throughout this book for your convenience in using the URL links with minimum keystrokes.

Some of your initial questions are probably about hCG itself.

Is hCG natural or synthetic?

Unless noted in the description as being produced by recombinant DNA, most brands are natural. For example, Novarel is manufactured by Ferring Pharmaceuticals, Inc. and Pregnyl is manufactured by Organon. Both brands are natural, derived from pregnant female urine, NOT from placenta, just as Dr. Simeons requires. A handy reference of many brand names of hCG, including manufacturers, is included in the table in the Ordering Information section of Step 14.

Are there any clinical studies on using this method of weight reduction?

Yes, these can be found at the following TinyURLs:

http://tinyurl.com/hcgstudy
Dr. Daniel Belluscio, Dr. Leonor Ripamonte, and Dr. Marcelo Wolansky
Utility of an Oral Presentation of hCG (human Choriogonadotropin) for the Management of Obesity: A Double-Blind Study

http://tinyurl.com/hcgstudy2
Daniel O. Belluscio M.D. and Leonor E. Ripamonte M.D.
Utility of an oral formulation of hCG for obesity treatment: A Double-Blind study

http://tinyurl.com/hcgstudy3
Leela S. Craig, Ruth E. Ray, Samuel H. Waxlerm, and Helen Madigan
Chorionic Gonadotropin in the Treatment of Obese Women
Am. J. Clinical Nutrition, Mar 1963; 12: 230 - 234.
A study that failed to reproduce good results using non-protocol foods and 550 calories.

http://tinyurl.com/hcgstudy4
A. T. Simeons
Chorionic Gonadotrophin in the Treatment of Obese Women
Am. J. Clinical Nutrition, Sep 1963; 13: 197 - 198.

Dr. Simeons' own rebuttal of the Craig study results.

http://tinyurl.com/hcgstudy5
Barry W. Frank
The Use of Chorionic Gonadotropin Hormone in the Treatment of Obesity A Double-Blind Study
Am. J. Clinical Nutrition, Mar 1964; 14: 133 - 136.
A study that concluded that hCG doesn't have significant impact on weight reduction, but used 200 IU and 1030 calories instead of doing the proper protocol.

http://tinyurl.com/hcgstudy6
James H. Hutton
The Use of Chorionic Gonadotropin in the Treatment of Obesity
Am. J. Clinical Nutrition, Feb 1965; 16: 277.
A Letter to the Editor explaining why the Frank study failed to get good results and affirming good results in Chicago using the original protocol.

http://tinyurl.com/hcgstudy7
A. T. W. Simeons
Chorionic Gonadotrophin in the Treatment of Obesity
Am. J. Clinical Nutrition, Sep 1964; 15: 188 - 190.
Dr. Simeons' own rebuttal of the Frank study results.

http://tinyurl.com/hcgstudy8
Harry A. Gusman
Chorionic Gonadotropin in Obesity: Further Clinical Observations
Am. J. Clinical Nutrition, Jun 1969; 22: 686 - 695.
A positive article based on clinical work with hCG and obesity, as well as explanations for why six studies failed to reproduce good results with hCG.

http://tinyurl.com/hcgstudy9
Margaret J. Albrink
Chorionic Gonadotropin and Obesity?
Am. J. Clinical Nutrition, Jun 1969; 22: 681 - 685.
A negative review of the Gusman article that found hCG to be effective in weight reduction.

http://tinyurl.com/hcgstudy10
James H. Hutton
Chorionic Gonadotropin and Obesity
Am. J. Clinical Nutrition, Mar 1970; 23: 243 - 244.
A Letter to the Editor refuting the Albrink article.

http://tinyurl.com/hcgstudy11
W. L. Asher and Harold W. Harper
Effect of human chorionic gonadotrophin on weight loss, hunger, and feeling of well-being
Am. J. Clinical Nutrition, Feb 1973; 26: 211 - 218.
An hCG study with positive results.

http://tinyurl.com/hcgstudy12
Jules Hirsch and Theodore B. Van Itallie

The treatment of obesity
Am. J. Clinical Nutrition, Oct 1973; 26: 1039 - 1041.
Letter refuting the Asher and Harper study results.

http://tinyurl.com/hcgstudy13
W. L. Asher and Harold W. Harper
Human chorionic gonadotropin treatment for obesity: a rebuttal
Am. J. Clinical Nutrition, May 1974; 27: 450 - 455.
Response to Hirsch and Vitallie's re-examination of their study.

http://tinyurl.com/hcgstudy14
M. R. Stein, R. E. Julis, C. C. Peck, W. Hinshaw, J. E. Sawicki, and J. J. Deller, Jr.
Ineffectiveness of human chorionic gonadotropin in weight reduction: a double-blind study
Am. J. Clinical Nutrition, Sep 1976; 29: 940 - 948.
An attempt to duplicate the Asher and Harper study that failed to do so.

http://tinyurl.com/hcgstudy15
P. Bradley
Human chorionic gonadotropin in weight reduction
Am. J. Clinical Nutrition, May 1977; 30: 649 – 654.
Letter to the Editor refuting the Stein study results.

http://tinyurl.com/hcgstudy16
M. R. Stein, R. E. Julis, C. C. Peck, W. Hinshaw, J. E. Sawicki, and J. J. Deller, Jr.
Human chorionic gonadotropin in weight reduction: a reply
Am. J. Clinical Nutrition, May 1977; 30: 652 - 653.
Rebuttal of Dr. Bradley's article.

No PDF available
M. R. Stein, R. E. Julis, C. C. Peck, W. Hinshaw, J. E. Sawicki, and J. J. Deller, Jr.
HCG clarification: a reply
Am. J. Clinical Nutrition, Jan 1978; 31: 3 - 4.

No PDF available
P. Bradley
HCG clarification
Am. J. Clinical Nutrition, Jan 1978; 31: 3 - 4.

http://tinyurl.com/hcgstudy17
G.A. Bray
Drug treatment of obesity
Am. J. Clinical Nutrition, Feb 1992; 55: 538S - 544S.
Mentions hCG negative studies in the Miscellaneous section.

http://tinyurl.com/hcgstudy18
Ezra Sohar
A Forty-Day—550 Calorie Diet in the Treatment of Obese Outpatients
Am. J. Clinical Nutrition, Sep 1959; 7: 514 - 518.
An hCG study that did not follow the exact protocol, but did get weight reduction results.

http://tinyurl.com/hcgstudy19
Ezra Sohar and Ephraim Sneh
Follow-up of obese patients: 14 years after a successful reducing diet
Am. J. Clinical Nutrition, Aug 1973; 26: 845 - 848.
Follow-up that showed that Sohar's group of hCG patients regained the weight in 14 years.

Before and after photos from a successful clinical study on hCG:
http://tinyurl.com/hcgstudy20

Another successful study with before and after photos:
http://tinyurl.com/hcgstudy21

This is a link to research that you can share with your doctor: http://tinyurl.com/hcgstudy22

Does hCG have any side effects or contraindications?

Yes, according to Dr. S beginning on page 42, brittle fingernails may become normal and professional singers may note an improvement in their voices. Blood pressure and blood sugar tends to normalize, cholesterol readings can become abnormally high, but with better ratios during treatment, only to become normal afterwards, and arthritis and rheumatism symptoms are lessened. Colitis, duodenal or gastric ulcers, varicose ulcers, certain allergies, psoriasis, loss of hair, brittle fingernails, and migraines, which can improve in pregnancy, can also improve during hCG treatment for obesity.

If you already have a tendency to have gall bladder issues or are genetically pre-disposed to gallbladder disease, the diet itself could aggravate that problem because there is little fat during the weight reduction portion of the protocol. Likewise, if you have gout, the diet could cause an aggravation of symptoms. Some people in my support group that had not been diagnosed with gout yet, were finally diagnosed and treated appropriately because the diet brought it out enough to be recognized for what it was by a doctor. With any drug there is the possibility of an allergic reaction or unusual reaction that may cause skin rash, difficulty breathing, collapse, or even death. No severe adverse reactions to hCG at these low doses have been experienced in my support group. hCG side effects listed on the package insert are for the prescribed dose for fertility treatments – which are at least 5,000 IU in one shot and can go up to 10,000 IU. It is unlikely that our extremely small dose would cause any of those symptoms. At the larger doses used for fertility treatments, the side effects and contraindications are listed at this link: **http://tinyurl.com/hcgwarnings** You may also check for drug interactions at this link: **http://tinyurl.com/hcginteraction**

Dr Simeons explains on pages 38-39 that "It is produced in enormous quantities, so that during certain phases of her pregnancy a woman may excrete as much as **one million International Units per day** in her urine...." How could a substance that is circulating in such large amounts during pregnancy be a significant risk to people? I think that to keep this in perspective, you must consider the dosage that is injected into our bodies during this diet is somewhere between 125 IU and 200 IU TOTAL, and that is NOT a level per ml of blood. Following are the pregnancy levels given in IU per ml of blood.

According to the Department of Obstetrics And Gynecology at the University of New Mexico, a pregnant woman produces a peak hCG level at about 10 weeks gestation, when the median hCG concentration in serum or plasma samples is near 60,000 mIU/ml. Wide variations are found in different subjects, however, with concentrations that can vary from 2,000 to 50,000 mIU/ml. See the chart below for ranges of levels at various stages of pregnancy:

Weeks from the Last Menstrual Period (LMP)	Amount of hCG in mIU/ml
3	5 - 50
4	3 - 426
5	19 - 7,340
6	1,080 - 56,500
7-8	7,650 - 229,000
9-12	25,700 - 288,000
13-16	13,300 - 254,000
17-24	4,060 - 165,400
25 - 40	3,640 - 117,000

The side effects for me have been reduced depression, increased libido, discovery of a new wardrobe in my own closet in the form of smaller items that I can wear again, better lab results when I have my checkups, an optimistic outlook and a new feeling of self-determination and control over my future that I haven't had for years. Additional hCG-associated phenomenon include softer skin and fewer PCOS and fibromyalgia symptoms, as well as wardrobe malfunctions in the form of too-large clothes no longer staying in place when I don't move to a smaller size in time.

One OB/GYN who uses this diet told me that when people ask if this is a healthy way to reduce, that the preferred response is to respond asking them in return if it is healthy to remain obese.

Everyone says that I am fat because I eat too much and move too little. Is that true?

No, not according to Dr Simeons and not according to one researcher who studied the causes of obesity for over five years. When reading this explanation, keep in mind that what we call the hypothalamus today, at the time that the following was written, was called the diencephalon.

Pages 21-22 of Pounds and Inches:
"It was therefore not unreasonable to suppose that the complex operation of storing and issuing fuel to the body might also be controlled by the diencephalon. It has long been known that the content of sugar - another form of fuel - in the blood depends on a certain nervous center in the diencephalon. When this center is destroyed in laboratory animals, they develop a condition rather similar to human stable diabetes. It has also long been known that the destruction of another diencephalic center produces a voracious appetite and a rapid gain in weight in animals which never get fat spontaneously.

The Fat-bank

Assuming that in man such a center controlling the movement of fat does exist, its function would have to be much like that of a bank. When the body assimilates from the intestinal tract more fuel than it needs at the moment, this surplus is deposited in what may be compared with a current account. Out of this account it can always be withdrawn as required. All normal fat reserves are in such a current account, and it is probable that a diencephalic center manages the deposits and withdrawals. When now, for reasons which will be discussed later, the deposits grow rapidly while small withdrawals become more frequent, a point may be reached which goes beyond the diencephalon's banking capacity. Just as a banker might suggest to a wealthy client that instead of accumulating a large and unmanageable current account he should invest his surplus capital, the body appears to establish a fixed deposit into which all surplus funds go but from which they can no longer be withdrawn by the procedure used in a current account. In this way the diencephalic "fat-bank" frees itself from all work which goes beyond its normal banking capacity. The onset of obesity dates from the moment the diencephalon adopts this labor-saving ruse. Once a fixed deposit has been established the normal fat reserves are held at a minimum, while every available surplus is locked away in the fixed deposit and is therefore taken out of normal circulation."

So using this same analogy, when the disease of obesity is set in motion, the diencephalon (hypothalamus) begins to put the fat in an abnormal fixed fat deposit that is similar to a long-term CD (certificate of deposit), which cannot be tapped easily for a withdrawal in the way that a current (checking) account or a normal fat deposit can. Therefore, it is much more difficult to reduce the abnormal fat deposits than it is to reduce the normal ones. With this mechanism in mind, Dr Simeons goes on to explain: "Whether obesity is caused by a marked inherited deficiency of the fat-center or by some entirely different diencephalic regulatory disorder, its insurgence obviously has nothing to do with overeating and in either case obesity is certain to develop regardless of dietary restrictions. In these cases any enforced food deficit is made up from essential fat reserves and normal structural fat, much to the disadvantage of the patient's general health."

Finally, Gary Taubes found that historical records show that obesity, rather than following prosperity, seemed to occur in improverished populations, most of which ate the cheaper sources of food that happened to be carbohydrate-rich, rather than fat or protein-rich. Few societies have chosen to subsist on large amounts of carbohydrates instead of fat and protein, other than those forced to do so by poverty. Or in the case of the United States, foolish enough to believe the nutritional recommendations of a government strongly influenced by the grain industry to recommend what amounts to a "finishing" diet given to livestock to fatten them for sale.

Gary uses the example of a starving family in which the mothers are overweight, but the younger children are malnourished. Everything that we know about the maternal instinct tells us that the mothers are NOT overeating to the detriment of their children's health. Something else is going on. Even though the mother and the child are both starving, the mother is overweight. In that particular society, females were the ones doing most of the manual labor, so a sedentary lifestyle cannot explain it. One possibility is that the mother is eating the wrong foods. Another is that her hypothalamus is damaged, but the child's is not yet because it is too young for the damage to have taken place yet. Regardless, it shows that it does not take a lot of calories and certainly not overeating to become fat.

http://tinyurl.com/GaryTaubes
http://tinyurl.com/GaryTaubes2
http://tinyurl.com/GaryTaubes3
http://tinyurl.com/GaryTaubes4
http://tinyurl.com/GaryTaubes5
http://tinyurl.com/GaryTaubes6

Why (and how) does this diet work?

Dr Simeons discovered the ability of hCG to release what he calls "fixed" or "abnormal" fat stores Into the bloodstream for use as fuel. The abnormal type of fat storage or "deposit" as he calls it, is not normally available to the body for fuel in an obese person, making it extremely difficult for someone who has the disease of obesity to reduce body weight. From pages 37-38 of Pounds and Inches:

"A woman may gain weight during pregnancy, but she never becomes obese in the strict sense of the word. Under the influence of the HCG which circulates in enormous quantities in her body during pregnancy, her diencephalic banking capacity seems to be unlimited, and abnormal fixed deposits are never formed. At confinement she is suddenly deprived of HCG, and her diencephalic fat-center reverts to its normal capacity. It is only then that the abnormally accumulated fat is locked away again in a fixed deposit. From that moment on she is suffering from obesity and is subject to all its consequences.

Pregnancy seems to be the only normal human condition in which the diencephalic fat-banking capacity is unlimited. It is only during pregnancy that fixed fat deposits can be transferred back into the normal current account and freely drawn upon to make up for any nutritional deficit. During pregnancy, every ounce of reserve fat is placed at the disposal of the growing fetus. Were this not so, an obese woman, whose normal reserves are already depleted, would have the greatest difficulties in bringing her pregnancy to full term. There is considerable evidence to suggest that it is the HCG produced in large quantities in the placenta which brings about this diencephalic change.

Though we may be able to increase the diencephalic fat banking capacity by injecting HCG, this does not in itself affect the weight, just as transferring monetary funds from a fixed deposit into a current account does not make a man any poorer; to become poorer it is also necessary that he freely spends the money which thus becomes available. In pregnancy the needs of the growing embryo take care of this to some extent, but in the treatment of obesity there is no embryo, and so a very severe dietary restriction must take its place for the duration of treatment.

Only when the fat which is in transit under the effect of HCG is actually consumed can more fat be withdrawn from the fixed deposits. In pregnancy it would be most undesirable if the fetus were offered ample food only when there is a high influx from the intestinal tract. Ideal nutritional conditions for the fetus can only be achieved when the mother's blood is continually saturated with food, regardless of whether she eats or not, as otherwise a period of starvation might hamper the steady growth of the embryo. It seems that HCG brings about this continual saturation of the blood, which is the reason why obese patients under treatment with HCG never feel hungry in spite of their drastically reduced food intake."

Isn't Kevin Trudeau a convicted criminal?

KT pleaded guilty to larceny in 1990 in Massachusetts after being charged with depositing $80,000 in worthless checks. In 1991, he pleaded guilty to credit-card fraud in federal district court and was sentenced to nearly two years in prison. He has paid his debt to society. The details are available for your reading pleasure at: **http://tinyurl.com/Trudeaupast.** Most of us in my support group found this protocol from seeing a Kevin Trudeau infomercial or buying his book in a store. I for one am eternally grateful that he brought this to the masses. He opened my mind to doing the research to find my diet support group and Dr. Simeons. However, when in doubt regarding this diet, the inventor, Dr. Simeons always rules.

Kevin has also had his troubles with the FTC because of his marketing practices on TV commercials, including the ones for the diet book: **http://tinyurl.com/Trudeauruling** As you can see, the FTC doesn't even have the correct hormone referenced, however. It would appear that the government can't be bothered with the facts about the diet.

In addition, the appeals court found that the fine and the ban were not imposed according to legal standards, further fueling the contention that the government is persecuting Kevin Trudeau and isn't even following the proper rules in order to do so: **http://tinyurl.com/Trudeauappeal**

Preparation for the Diet

So many times, I have had people ask me, "Please, take me through this diet, step by step, in order." So I decided to organize this book in just that way. Each section of this book will be based on a part of the diet, beginning with preparing for the diet (which is at least half the battle), then releasing the weight, going on to stabilizing the new weight, and next, maintaining the weight. I will discuss in chronological order, the steps involved in each part of the diet. This first section contains all of the steps for preparing for doing the diet.

Step 1 – Read this book in its entirety.

You need to have in your mind the "big picture" of how this is going to work and what you will be doing. Picture yourself successfully doing each of the parts of the diet.

Step 2 – Take a "before" picture of yourself.

Yes, it is humbling, but you will be glad that you did it later, when it is time for a side-by-side comparison of your before and after photos. Sometimes, we forget how things were, once they have changed, which is referred to as the "apex" effect. Sometimes, we can't see the changes that have happened and we need others to tell us what changes they see as our bodies change, becoming slender and trim. The photos along the way help to record those changes so that we can acknowledge them, even if it requires asking someone else to look at them and tell us specifically what they see in the way of changes.

Step 3 – Take your "before" measurements.

Again, later you will be happy that you did. Continue measuring with the same tape measure throughout your hCG adventure. To take my measurements, I am using a gadget called an Accu-Measure Myo Tape Measure that makes it easier if you don't have anyone living with you to help you. I've assembled for you many products that are helpful on this diet protocol, including this one, in one place: **www.hcgdietingstore.com** Whether you purchase from this site or not, the photos and descriptions should help you to find these helpful items.

Step 4 – Read Dr. Simeons' "Pounds and Inches" all the way through.

Take some notes or highlight passages if something strikes a chord with you. It's a short read and quite interesting for the most part. The time that you devote to do this will be invaluable.

Where can I find the original manuscript of Dr. Simeons' book?

The Weight Loss Cure "They" Don't Want You to Know About by Kevin Trudeau is based on a much older manuscript from 1971 called *Pounds and Inches: A New Approach to Obesity* written by Albert Theodore William (A.T.W.) Simeons, M.D., a British doctor who had a clinic in Rome. Dr S started prescribing the hCG diet in 1955, because in Pounds and Inches, dated 1971, he mentions twice that he began it 16 years ago. He also mentions that he had been studying obesity for 40 years, so it took him 24 years of research to develop his innovative theories on the origins of and treatment for obesity. KT decided to add Phases 1 and 4 and made other adjustments to "update" it for current conditions that did not exist in 1971, such as the need for eating organic food and avoiding additives.

A scanned copy of the original *Pounds and Inches* book by Dr. Simeons is available at: **http://tinyurl.com/PoundsandInches** for comparison and reference. You can see that it is not

OCR'd. It is a photocopy of the bound book and therefore is the real ORIGINAL. Most of my support group members follow one of these versions of the protocol and food list (Trudeau or Simeons), but some follow a particular clinic's protocol and food list instead.

What are the Phases? I don't see them in the Simeons manuscript.

There are four Phases that were added by KT in his book. They did not exist in Dr. Simeons' manuscript as such. Dr S only explains what to do during hCG administration and what to do for three weeks after, corresponding to KT Phases 2 and 3, along with instructing to add sugar and starch back into your diet very gradually, which corresponds to Phase 4.

o Phase 1 – KT believes that our bodies are toxic now and need cleansing for 30 days or longer before the cure. See: **http://tinyurl.com/60steps**
o Phase 2 – Dr. Simeons' hCG plus diet administration protocol as described in his manuscript.
o Phase 3 – The first 3 weeks after your last 500 calorie day, which is 72 hours after your last dose of hCG. This is CRUCIAL as this is the part that stabilizes your weight setpoint at the new level. You are to have no sugar or starches and weigh every morning to make sure that you haven't gained more than 2 pounds above your LIW (Last Injection Weight) or LSDW (Last Sublingual Dose Weight), or 2 pounds less. Steak days are used if you go above the 2 pounds; if you go below the 2 pounds, you must eat more calories to return to within 2 pounds of the LIW or LSDW.
o Phase 4 – After the first three weeks and beyond, you can add sugar and starch very gradually, then eat normally after the gradual changes, but you must weigh every morning and adjust your intake the next day if you have gained. I personally feel you will gain again unless you avoid food additives and concentrate on non-toxic, homemade, organic if you can afford it, food and products.

Do I have to do all of Kevin's MUST DO's?

Please don't let KT's list of "MUST DO's" stand in your way of using this diet. They are really not MUSTs at all. If I had thought that I had to do everything in KT's book, I would have said to myself, "Well, that's just not going to work for me. I can't afford to even try this diet plan." In fact, I found that it is affordable and easily can be done on a middle-class income, especially when you consider that less food is needed while on Phase 2. The reduced food expenses can pay for the hCG sometimes.

That being said, although you don't need to follow all of KT'S recommendations and still will lose weight, going back to eating and doing exactly the same things that put on the pounds is highly likely to cause the same conditions that contributed to the onset of obesity to occur again. I suggest trying some of it, particularly the switch to organic foods and avoiding food additives such as MSG, artificial sweeteners, and high fructose corn syrup. See those sections in other parts of this book for information about the reasons that these are likely to be health concerns.

Should I have blood tests run before starting the diet?

Many doctors and clinics require them and it might afford you some peace of mind that you don't have a condition that needs attention. If you're looking for an inexpensive resource for getting a full "before" blood work-up, **http://www.lef.org/bloodtest/** offers a complete blood panel. "Chemistry Profile and Complete Blood Count" is number 6 on the list of products, and the price is $35 for members ($75 membership) or $47 for non-members. Another source for a CBC is: **http://www.directlabs.com/**

Can I just do this plan a few days a week?

Are you trying to fit this diet into your life, or fit your life into the diet? You must give this diet first priority in order to be successful. You will never know what improved results that you could have achieved doing this diet exactly as written if you don't do it that way.

One of the members of my support group, M Paige, answered this question in these awesome words: "I'm wondering what you're feeling that motivated you to ask a question like that? I know the program looks very restrictive (and in many ways it is) and you may be thinking NO WAY could I do that consistently for 43 days. I think it's a fair question, because the key to success of any kind, be it personal, professional, or in this case, health-related, stems from the ability to be consistent. And if you're like me, you've **been** consistent before and seen **NO results**. And you have probably also been consistent before and seen only **temporary** results. So, in light of past experiences, maybe you're feeling like you can't (psychologically) take another let down. Maybe you feel like you're tired of being **gung-ho** about one more diet that you figure doesn't work in the long term. Maybe you're tired of getting all wound up and psyched up for something **again** without the long term outcome you want. Whatever it is. I think most of us probably understand you at that exact level.

BUT, all that being said, I will say this to you about this particular plan: The HCG diet is not easy but it is simple. If you decide to do it, and do it properly, you will learn so much about yourself, you'll have **no doubt** that your results will be permanent. It's about **way more** than losing weight. You will discover that as you go. You'll notice that LOTS of deeply seated emotional issues and dependency issues come to the forefront. It is precisely because of the calorie restriction and the commitment to stay true to the protocol that many of us must deal with the issues for which we'd normally use food to mood-alter ourselves. But I learned and came to terms with the new role of food in my life. We're all finding better and different coping skills to deal with a hectic and stress-filled world. As we get closer to mastering these skills after just a few weeks on the protocol, we **know** in our deepest beings, that we will never go back to being obese again. EVER. We just know. You can have that, too.

But if you give yourself a few days off every week, you not only won't get the physical result that you desire, but also, and worse, you won't ever reach that place emotionally that will free you from using food to mood-alter. I hope you continue to consider it carefully. I think your question was legitimate. But I also think it's an indication of fear of failure (Can I really do this?!?) and possibly some concern over having to let go of something as wonderful and meaningful and dependable (displaced as it is) as food has been for some of us, in terms of comfort and stress relief. Think it over. Carefully. This is a life-changing protocol. Those who start should be prepared for all the changes it will bring, both physical and emotional."

I have to agree – totally.

Does the weight stay off?

I'll answer that by stating that I have had no problems whatsoever keeping the weight off in Phases 3 and 4 so far. I am not at my goal weight yet, but what I have taken off so far has stayed off with little effort. I'm eating a lot more than I used to be able to without gaining. And if I do gain one day, I cut out sugar and starch the next day, and the weight falls right back off. THAT never happened for me before.

I am not overweight, but my body is not shaped the way I want. Will this work for me?

This is a good protocol for anyone with abnormal fat deposits. Even people who only need to lose 15 to 20 pounds can use hCG to reshape. Dr. Simeons describes this in the manuscript in the section about the emaciated lady on page 32.

When does the hypothalamus reset to heal?

KT's book made it sound as though the hypothalamus (formerly called the diencephalon) resets in P3. However, I espouse a theory that two "resetting" events need to happen. First, the hypothalamus needs to regain its former ability to bank fat properly and not excessively or in fixed (abnormal, hard to access and release) deposits as it did in the past. I think that this also affects your appetite and satiety, making you feel satisfied with less and realizing when you don't want more food.

From Pounds and Inches, page 93: "Most patients hardly ever need to skip a meal. If they have eaten a heavy lunch they feel no desire to eat their dinner, and in this case no increase takes place. If they keep their weight at the point reached at the end of the treatment, even a heavy dinner does not bring about an increase of two pounds on the next morning and does not therefore call for any special measures. Most patients are surprised how small their appetite has become and yet how much they can eat without gaining weight. They no longer suffer from an abnormal appetite and feel satisfied with much less food than before. In fact, they are usually disappointed that they cannot manage their first normal meal, which they have been planning for weeks."

This change in the hypothalamus, I believe, happens in P2, after 21 days on VLCD+hCG. Here is my evidence from what Dr S said in P & I, page 51:

"We never give a treatment lasting less than 26 days, even in patients needing to lose only 5 pounds. **It seems that even in the mildest cases of obesity the diencephalon requires about three weeks rest from the maximal exertion to which it has been previously subjected in order to regain fully its normal fat-banking capacity.** Clinically this expresses itself, in the fact that, when in these mild cases, treatment is stopped as soon as the weight is normal, which may be achieved in a week, it is much more easily regained than after a full course of 23 injections."

If that doesn't sound like the hypothalamus resetting during Phase 2, I don't know what does. If you cheat, your extremely low caloric dietary intake is not taking the place of a fetus and the hypothalamus does not get that rest. For that reason, it seems prudent to be particularly vigilant with regard to NOT cheating during the first 21 days of the VLCD or 21 subsequent sequential back-to-back days sometime during the VLCD.

I refer to this event as the hypothalamus resetting.

However, to avoid creating the conditions under which obesity happened originally, the avoidance of starch and sugar for an additional three weeks, plus steak days if the weight increases more than 2 pounds, in what KT calls Phase 3, is also necessary to stabilize your setpoint at the lowered weight, according to Dr. Simeons. Keeping the weight steadily between two pounds over or under the LIW resets the body's weight setpoint so that your body tends to stay near the LIW from then on, I believe.

I refer to that event as resetting your body's weight setpoint.

Step 5 – Apply to join the HCG Diet Made Simple support group.

Apply to join the HCG Diet Made Simple support group by sending an email to: HCGDietMadeSimple-subscribe@yahoogroups.com. Posting daily will help you to keep good records, get support and encouragement, and help you to be accountable every day.

My best advice to anyone who reads this book is to read and follow the food list in the Simeons manuscript. You should get success that way. If someone says that they eat blueberries and still lose and you want to try that, please realize that you do so at your own risk. Remember, your mileage may vary.

Step 6 – Take stock of your personal readiness state.

Answer the following questions for yourself:
- o Can you commit to staying on the program for the time needed?
- o How easily can you fit the program into your lifestyle?
- o What opposition will you have from family and friends?
- o What support will you have from family and friends?
- o Will you have the support and help of your doctor?
- o Will you be confident enough to do the program on your own, or do you need to use a clinic to provide you with meds and support?
- o Do you have the financial means to purchase the needed supplies?
- o Do you have the time needed to complete at least one round?
- o Are you ready to change your life?

Step 7 – Decide if you need a new scale to weigh your body.

Decide if you need a new scale to weigh your body. Many models now have body fat readings, which while not as accurate as other methods, can at least show you a long-term trend. Just don't freak out if it appears to go up sometimes. Those scales depend on level of hydration and can measure differently within an hour of the last measurement of body fat. Only a Bod Pod measurement is reliable.

Step 8 – Read "Pounds and Inches" AGAIN!!!

You will be surprised at what you notice that you missed the first time. I have read it hundreds of times now.

Can my teenaged son or daughter do this diet?

Anyone past puberty is probably old enough to do this diet. Dr B's clinical study included teenagers as young as 15. Dr. S treated teenagers and this is what he states on page 54 about that: "While on the question of menstruation it must be added that in teenaged girls the period may in some rare cases be delayed and exceptionally stop altogether." Dr S apparently even treated those as young as 11. From his rebuttal letter in the American Journal of Clinical Nutrition, Vol. 13, September 1963: "On analyzing the case sheets we found that the group was composed of 122 males and 378 females who ranged in age from **eleven** to seventy-eight years." **http://tinyurl.com/hcgstudy4**

Can I do this diet if I am vegetarian?

Dr. S states that vegetarians will lose about half as much weight per day as meat-eaters, but he does give the alternatives of low-fat cottage cheese or three egg whites with one whole egg, if fish as well as meat is not eaten (p. 63). My dear friend Shalom, whom you may have seen on the Mike and Juliet Show segment on hCG (**http://tinyurl.com/MikeandJuliet1 http://tinyurl.com/MikeandJuliet2**

http://tinyurl.com/MikeandJuliet3), formulated a successful way to do this diet vegan. Her website, www.hcgcoach.com, is extremely helpful for vegetarian alternatives for this diet.

Step 9 – Approach your doctor about the protocol, if you choose.

Determine whether your doctor will be supportive by monitoring your changes in labwork values or actually will prescribe the hCG for you.

What if my doctor doesn't agree?

I'll bet the good doctor would tell people to have surgery instead of hCG. Or just tell folks to push away from the table and move more, as if that works for everyone, which it certainly does NOT. If "eat less, exercise more" worked, or even if "calories in = calories out" or "a calorie is a calorie" was true, the US would not be the fattest nation in the world right now. We have been told wrong, plain and simple.

The USDA Food Pyramid, used from 1992-2005, which recommended eating more grain than any other food group (6 to 11 servings a day), is to blame for a lot of this. Haven't you ever heard the term "grain-finished" when referring to cattle or other livestock? That's what they do to fatten up livestock. Any farmer could tell you that.

A superb writer that spent at least five years of research to determine what was helping to cause the obesity epidemic agrees with me about this: **http://tinyurl.com/GaryTaubes**

A Florida physician who is a former head of Harvard's Nutrition department agrees with me: **http://tinyurl.com/Willix**

One of the other biggest problems is that we have so many food additives, such as MSG and high fructose corn syrup, in almost everything that you can buy in a bottle, can, or box in a grocery store. MSG is what is used to create lesions on the hypothalamus to make mice obese for lab experiments. Ask any scientist.

The answer is to stop eating this way and use hCG to help your hypothalamus to heal that damage that makes us hungry and obese.

Step 11 – If your doctor will not support you, review the Clinics section of the book.

If your doctor will not support you, review the Clinics section of the book to decide if a clinic is for you.

Step 12 – Decide whether to use a clinic or go it on your own.

Decide whether to use a clinic or go it on your own. Keep in mind that clinics make more money the longer that it takes you to lose the weight, so they would therefore have a vested interest in changing the original protocol to ensure that you lose weight more slowly, although not so slowly that you would stop using them. Many of the clinics do little more than requiring and checking initial lab work. Then you are given instructions and you are on your own for a much higher price than you would pay to do this yourself. It would be a rare clinic nowadays that would follow your health very closely during your weight reduction. If you do find one that will, it might be worth the extra money because you can't put a price on your health if you have many pre-existing conditions that you want monitored.

Is there anyone with a past heart attack using hCG successfully without problems?

Here is exactly what Dr. Simeons says on page 87:
"The Heart
Disorders of the heart are not as a rule contraindications. In fact, the removal of abnormal fat - particularly from the heart-muscle and from the surrounding of the coronary arteries - can only be beneficial in cases of myocardial weakness, and many such patients are referred to us by cardiologists. Within the first week of treatment all patients - not only heart cases - remark that they have lost much of their breathlessness

Coronary Occlusion
In obese patients who have recently survived a coronary occlusion, we adopt the following procedure in collaboration with the cardiologist. We wait until no further electrocardiographic changes have occurred for a period of three months. Routine treatment is then started under careful control and it is usual to find a further electrocardiographic improvement of a condition which was previously stationary.

In the thousands of cases we have treated we have not once seen any sort of coronary incident occur during or shortly after treatment. The same applies to cerebral vascular accidents. Nor have we ever seen a case of thrombosis of any sort develop during treatment, even though a high blood pressure is rapidly lowered. In this respect, too, the HCG treatment resembles pregnancy."

Could my gall bladder problems act up while on hCG?

According to Dr. S, "Small stones in the gall bladder may in patients who have recently had typical colics cause more frequent colics under treatment with HCG. This may be due to the almost complete absence of fat from the diet, which prevents the normal emptying of the gall bladder. Before undertaking treatment we explain to such patients that there is a risk of more frequent and possibly severe symptoms and that it may become necessary to operate. If they are prepared to take this risk and provided they agree to undergo an operation if we consider this imperative, we proceed with treatment, as after weight reduction with HCG the operative risk is considerably reduced in an obese patient. In such cases we always give a drug which stimulates the flow of bile, and in the majority of cases nothing untoward happens. On the other hand, we have looked for and not found any evidence to suggest that the HCG treatment leads to the formation of gallstones as pregnancy sometimes does." p. 87

Can diabetics use this diet?

Dr. S states on page 43: "In an obese patient suffering from a fairly advanced case of stable diabetes of many years duration in which the blood sugar may range from 300-400 mg, it is often possible to stop all anti-diabetes medication after the first few days of treatment. The blood sugar continues to drop from day to day and often reaches normal values in 2-3 weeks. As in pregnancy, this phenomenon is not observed in the brittle type of diabetes, and as some cases that are predominantly stable may have a small brittle factor in their clinical makeup, all obese diabetics have to be kept under a very careful and expert watch. A brittle case of diabetes is primarily due to the inability of the pancreas to produce sufficient insulin, while in the stable type, diencephalic regulations seem to be of greater importance. That is possibly the reason why the stable form responds so well to the HCG method of treating obesity, whereas the brittle type does not. Obese patients are generally suffering from the stable type, but a stable type may gradually change into a brittle one, which is usually associated with a loss of weight. Thus, when an obese diabetic finds that he is losing weight without diet or treatment, he should at once have his diabetes expertly attended to. There is some evidence to suggest that the change from stable to brittle is more liable to occur in patients who are taking insulin for their stable diabetes."

Health Improvements

Many hCG dieters in my support group have reported various improvements in their health, such as stabilized blood sugar, lowered blood pressure, more energy, reduced body fat percentage, reduced BMI to normal, and have been able to discontinue medications after releasing weight with hCG.

hCG and Cancer Prevention/Treatment

Someone might try to alarm you by saying that hCG is a cancer marker. Please get the facts. hCG is a cancer marker for gestational trophoblastic tumors and some germ cell cancers, and for males, who would not normally have hCG in any amount, because hCG is secreted by some of those cancer tumors. However, that does NOT mean that having hCG in your system is a bad thing, or all pregnant women would be afraid that their pregnancy would give them cancer. Can you imagine? The truth is that hCG is also used to TREAT cancer: **http://tinyurl.com/cancerstudy1**

Human chorionic gonadotropin (HCG) induction of apoptosis in breast cancer.
Definition of Apoptosis: A form of cell death in which a programmed sequence of events leads to the elimination of cells without releasing harmful substances into the surrounding area.
http://tinyurl.com/cancerstudy2

Scientists at the Massey Cancer Center at Virginia Commonwealth University have validated prior laboratory research showing the efficacy of human chorionic gonadotropin (hCG) in treating cancer. Using prostate cancer cell lines, hCG was shown to radiosensitize cancer cells as well as facilitate apoptosis, or normal cell death. **http://tinyurl.com/cancerstudy3**

Prior work by Milkhaus Laboratory yielded similar results for breast cancer cell lines.
http://tinyurl.com/cancerstudy4

Newsweek November 4, 1996 AIDS' Achilles' heel? (pregnancy hormone 'human chorionic gonadotropin' found to eliminate Kaposi's sarcoma) **http://tinyurl.com/cancerstudy5**
http://tinyurl.com/cancerstudy6
http://tinyurl.com/cancerstudy7
http://tinyurl.com/cancerstudy8
http://tinyurl.com/cancerstudy9
http://tinyurl.com/cancerstudy10
http://tinyurl.com/cancerstudy11
http://tinyurl.com/cancerstudy12
http://tinyurl.com/cancerstudy13
http://tinyurl.com/cancerstudy14
http://tinyurl.com/cancerstudy15
http://tinyurl.com/cancerstudy16
http://tinyurl.com/cancerstudy17
http://tinyurl.com/cancerstudy18
http://tinyurl.com/cancerstudy19
http://tinyurl.com/cancerstudy20

Health improvements reported by some of the folks in my support group include blood pressure improving from 145/91 before hCG to 120/82 afterwards and from 150/110 to 118/70 (using salt!). Body fat reduction from 28% to 18% and BMI from 33 to 27 are other changes that people are seeing.

Step 13 – Choose a clinic, if needed.

My observation about many clinics is that few follow a strict Simeons hCG diet protocol. Many recommend ways of doing the diet that prolong the treatment period by reducing the rapidity of weight release, perhaps for obvious reasons that they will make more money the longer that it takes you.

Clinic Comparisons

TWE HCG Solutions
http://tinyurl.com/clinic1
A clinic recommended by KT that allows you to go to any of 1700 labs across the nation to do advance blood work, reviews the labs, and then prescribes the hCG for you to administer to yourself.

Daniel Oscar Belluscio, M.D.

The hCG Obesity and Research Clinic in Argentina has been using a sublingual formula with over 8,000 patients. To see results that he has gotten: **http://tinyurl.com/clinicB**

Interestingly, Dr B has two new patents filed on hCG, one for an "oral" (sublingual) administration method and one for using it to treat mood disorders and alcoholism: **http://tinyurl.com/BPatent** **http://tinyurl.com/BPatent2**

Millennium Day Spa (Releana)

http://tinyurl.com/clinic3 provides sublingual hCG through affiliated doctors.

Transformations Medical Weight Loss
http://tinyurl.com/clinic4

Weight Control of Texas

http://tinyurl.com/clinic5 will give you shots to do at home. They have been doing this for 35 years, but 15 years ago made a couple of changes to Dr. Simeons' protocol. Instead of injecting 6 days out of the week, you only inject M-W-F with 250 IU and instead of 500 calories per day, you eat 750 calories. The clinic nurse said that everyone loses the same amount of weight as they would with the daily injections and 500 calories per day. I have not been able to verify that this assertion is true with any group members that have gone to this clinic. My concern with this is because Dr S specifically said on page 86: "Any attempt to economize in time by giving larger doses at longer intervals is doomed to produce less satisfactory results."

The Weight Loss Solution

http://tinyurl.com/clinic6 is a chiropractic practice providing hCG through a partnership with a doctor.

Lufkin Health and Wellness
http://tinyurl.com/clinic9

Quick Clinic Comparison Chart

Differences/Clinics	NHW (Now Defunct)	TWE (formerly known as GHI)	Transformations	Releana
Cost of hCG	Premixed injections, The start up fee and talking to Kathy and Noka anytime is $149.00. The first six week protocol is $426.50. Anything past that is $59/week plus $28.50 per shipment (whether it's one week or six). One person reports $711 total for a 10-week round, including the required lab.	Premixed injections, $305 for 6 weeks	$50 a week for hCG and appetite suppressants $25 a week for hCG only	Premixed Sublingual, $250 for 30 days
Cost of Required Labs	Cost of a CBC panel	$250 labs and $200 doc review	$130	Unknown
Freeze hCG?	Yes	Yes	No, they don't even state to refrigerate.	No, but they do state to refrigerate.
Brand of hCG	Novarel	Abraxis	Unknown	Unknown

Quick Program Comparison Chart

Differences/ Programs	Simeons	Trudeau	NHW	NWE/GHI	Transformations	Releana
Calories per day allowed	500	500	800, three day load, or load for two days, then take one day off (still eating anything) then begin daily shots again, different food plan.	No food plan, you eat what you want.	800, No load, different food plan with fat free foods, processed foods, margarine, and artificial sweeteners. NO coffee or tea. Also, they allow 1 can of diet soda a day, and frozen yogurt.	No-calorie drinks, 3.5-oz lean protein for lunch and dinner, a 3.5-oz serving of approved vegetable for lunch and a different one for dinner, 2 approved fruits per day. No starch, sugar or fat of any kind.
Grissini/Melba	Yes	No	No	Yes	Yes	No
Oranges	Yes	No	Yes	Yes	Yes	Yes
Shellfish	Yes	No	Yes	Yes	Yes	Yes
Broccoli/ Cauliflower/ Zucchini	No	No	Yes	Yes	Yes	Yes
Mix Vegetables	No	No, major typo in first edition	Two per meal	Yes	Yes	Yes
Organic	No	Yes	No	No	No	No
Cleanses	No	Yes	No	No	No	No
Skip a Day	Yes	Yes	Yes, two days	No	Yes, two days	No
Daily Dose	125IU	175-200IU	175IU	250IU	125IU	166IU twice
Stop During Period	Yes	Yes	Yes	Yes	No	No
Administration method	IM injection	IM injection	SC/SQ injection	SC/SQ injection	SC/SQ injection	Sublingual
Per Course Loss Limit	34 lbs or 40 lbs if obese	None	None	None	None	None
Per Course Day Limit	40 injections	40 injections	52 injections	40 injections	40 injections	None
Break length	6 weeks 8 weeks 12 weeks, etc.	3 weeks	2 weeks	2 weeks	3 weeks	None

Step 14 – If doing this without a clinic or physician, choose administration method and dosage, then place orders.

If doing this without a clinic or physician:
- o Decide whether to do Subcutaneous or Intramuscular injections OR use a sublingual mixture.
- o Determine how much hCG you will need to lose the weight you want.
  1. What dosage will you take?
  2. How many rounds do you need to do?
  3. Will other family or friends be doing the program with you?
- o Review the hCG suppliers section of the book and decide where to order hCG.
- o Order hCG.
- o Review the book sections for your chosen administration method and determine what supplies for giving injections or mixing sublingual that you need to purchase.
- o Order supplies.

What method of hCG administration should I use?

Some use intramuscular (IM) injections and some prefer subcutaneous (SC sometimes referred to as SQ) shots. Some use sublingual (SL) under the tongue. Some pharmacies have developed a nasal spray that could work in the same way as sublingual, through the blood vessels close to the surface in the thin internal lining of the nose. This is available through Dr. Morgan Jennie Titus N.D., Naturopath, 207-872-5450. Everyone has to choose which way they prefer, based on what works for them. Dr. Simeons suggested only IM, but many of us have found equal success using SC and SL. I have tried all three and believe that they all work equally well when done properly. Some doctors do think that the hCG degrades somewhat before reaching the bloodstream when using SQ, because it goes into the fat layer first, so dosage might need to be increased to compensate. SL is dosed twice a day rather than once and at higher dosage in order to compensate for reduced absorption and faster elimination.

A couple of other administration methods are being used by some, but I have experienced neither, because each has potential to be non-effective, according to my research. One method is transdermal hCG cream or gel. The concern that I have with this method is the size of the hCG molecule. For example, you must consider the difference in molecular weight between estrogen (272 to 296 Daltons), and hCG, which has a much larger molecule, (9500 to 40000 Daltons). I have serious concerns about the expected absorption transdermally of hCG for this reason. Only a limited number of drugs such as estrogen, testosterone, scopolomine, clonidine, and nitroglycerine, will fit the molecular weight, lipophilicity, and potency requirements for transdermal absorption. See **http://tinyurl.com/transdermal** for a discussion of transdermal delivery history.

Molecular weight table: **http://tinyurl.com/mwtable**
Table 1 summarizes the structure of the key hCG-related molecules. These vary in size from a molecular weight of 9500 (b-core fragment) to approximately 40000 (hyperglycosylated hCG).

Methods to enable large molecules to penetrate through the skin: **http://tinyurl.com/transpatent**
http://tinyurl.com/transmethods

I had also found a product, but it appears to be discontinued; no doubt you can guess the reason: **http://tinyurl.com/transdisc**

One of the members of my support group said that several neighbors went on the hCG Diet at the same time, with some using injections, some the nasal spray, and some the transdermal cream or gel from a pharmacy in New Jersey called Pharmacy Creations. The results are in: best weight reduction occurred with injections, with the nasal spray putting in a credible performance, with almost as much as the shots, and the cream trailed in at dead last. Based on all of this information, I doubt if it works. The future patches with batteries and all sound like they could work, but perhaps only locally rather than systemically.

Without some agent to increase absorption through skin, you could not get enough hCG in your system, I don't believe. The absorption-enhancing agent could be liposomes, dermal penetration enhancers, and lipophilic solvents and formulations, but the only thing that I seen that might accomplish this effectively is some patents for using lasers, ultrasound, or electrical current to make the skin more porous so that high molecular weight peptides like hCG can be absorbed through skin and then you might have to bathe in it and then use those methods to get systemic response.

One sustained-release form of HCG is a transdermal HCG patch, created like the fentanyl patch. In U.S. Patents No. 4,878,892, No. 4,940,456, No. 5,032,109, No. 5,158,537, and No. 5,250,023, transdermal delivery of proteins similar to hCG has been attained under the influence of an electric field, called iontophoretically or electroosmotically. Passive transdermal delivery is not effective for high-molecular-weight polypeptides and proteins, according to these patents, at least at not at therapeutically effective rates.

Dr Belluscio mentions in his double-blind study that the entire hCG molecule probably is not absorbed sublingually, either (even though we know that it works just the same), although I would think sublingual would allow absorbing a larger molecule than normal skin because you don't have the thick skin layer to get through between the blood vessels and the surface under the tongue.

The other method that I have concerns and unanswered questions about is "homeopathic" hCG. Please, if you are using this method, read this section without becoming defensive. As are all homeopathic remedies, this is diluted to the point that no actual hCG is left in the water and it is being called "homeopathic". However, it does not follow the classical homeopathic Law of Similars. Don't get me wrong; I think that classical homeopathy can work, but this does not follow the "First Law", which is that a substance that can cause a condition in a healthy person can also cure it in a person ill with that disease if it is diluted in that manner. hCG does NOT cause obesity in a healthy person, so it cannot work as a homeopathic remedy to cure it, according to the "First Law". Again, if you choose to use this product and are happy with it, I do not dispute your opinion, but I do have my own, based on research with an open mind, but not open so wide that I allow my brain to fall out in the process. I will even include the instructions for optimal implementation for this method, though I personally will not use it.

From Mediral, a company that MAKES the "homeopathic" hCG, comes this newsletter statement: "Mediral recommends that users of homeopathic hCG exercise prudence when counseling with clients to avoid making claims that the FTC might interpret as fraudulent or deceptive. There are, as yet, no monographs or provings of hCG. Do not claim the same results from homeopathic hCG that the prescription injectable hCG produces. The custom singular that Mediral makes of hCG is labeled 'HCG Detox' as a reminder that the only defensible use for homeopathic hCG is as a detoxifier."
http://tinyurl.com/hhcgdisclaimer

I think that the preceding statements speak for themselves. In fact, to me, they speak volumes. Both a naturopathic physician and a medical doctor that I have asked about "homeopathic" hormones stated that they do not exist and that there is no basis for believing that they would work. I mean, think about this: would you take "homeopathic" insulin (if it existed) with not even one molecule of insulin in it, if you were an insulin-dependent diabetic? I sure wouldn't. And you might want to think about why "homeopathic" insulin does not exist, if you think that "homeopathic" hormones are a good idea.

If you were infertile, would you trust "homeopathic" hCG to trigger your ovulation? No one that I know that wants the best chance of having a baby would. Would you trust your birth control to a "homeopathic" version of your oral contraceptive and risk potential failure of it, resulting in pregnancy? What about to protect your daughter from an unplanned pregnancy? If you wouldn't trust your blood sugar levels (and your life, potentially) or your reproductive control to it, why take that chance with your weight reduction and normalizing of your hypothalamic function? Isn't your healthy hypothalamus just as important? Isn't the possibility of healing your hypothalamus of the abnormal fat storage tendency worth using the same hCG that Dr Simeons used?

Please, if you do decide to try the "homeopathic", if you start to show signs of starvation, abandon it. Yes, that "homeopathic" hCG can be cheaper and easier to obtain than real hCG, though some companies are charging more than prescription hCG for the "homeopathic" and some are not even disclosing that it is not prescription. Many of the folks that I've spoken to that bought it were surprised to learn that it will not register a positive on a pregnancy test as real hCG will when drops of it are put on one. It does not need refrigeration, making it more convenient in many ways, but are you willing to trade the best results for convenience? It would be much easier, less controversial, and much more convenient for me to recommend the "homeopathic hCG drops", but I have to live with myself and look in the mirror each morning. Would it be worth it to potentially risk people's health by recommending to them that they do a 500 calorie diet without the benefit of real hCG that I KNOW will release at least 2000 calories from abnormal fat stores into their bloodstreams to keep them nourished and healthy? Not for me. Therefore, I have not risked trying or recommending either of these two methods (transdermal or "homeopathic") because I want to know that I am receiving real hCG at the proper dosage so that I have the best chance of receiving all of the potential benefits of hCG.

And I want you to have that opportunity, too.

What is OraThin?

OraThin is NOT a product that Kevin Trudeau recommends, nor is www.naturalcuresstore.com a Kevin Trudeau site. OraThin is NOT real hCG and therefore, obviously could not have exactly the same effects. It is marketed as an oral alternative to hCG. The ingredients can be verified at **http://tinyurl.com/OTingredients** where they also make negative statements about hCG having dangerous side effects, but they do not back up those statements with any clinical studies or other documentation. Clearly, they would have a vested interest in convincing you NOT to use real hCG because they want you to use their pills that don't have hCG in them. These products ship with a pamphlet titled: The Alternative hCG Weight Loss Protocol Inspired By: A.T.W Simeons M.D.

Which syringes/needles are used for hCG weight reduction shots?

The type of needle to use depends on whether you are doing subcutaneous (SC or SQ) or intramuscular (IM) hCG shots. The larger the gauge number, the smaller the needle's diameter. For example, a 21 gauge needle is thicker than a 29 gauge needle. More information is in the table entitled "Comparison of Injection Methods" in this section.

Which kind of injection should I use?

Dr. Simeons used intramuscular (IM), but some people report success with subcutaneous (SC or SQ) as well. Following are several clinical studies that show the findings about the differences. Part of these studies is a measurement of hCG levels in follicular fluid, which is a fertility treatment issue and not something we're concerned with for weight reduction. Blood (serum or plasma) levels and bioavailability are the most important things for us.

For drugs such as epinephrine, which need to be absorbed quickly if someone is having a severe allergic reaction, IM in the thigh has been proven to give the highest level of plasma concentration of epinephrine.

In a study specifically done with hCG, they injected both obese and non-obese women with hCG. They first gave everyone subcutaneous injections, and 4 weeks later gave them IM injections. They found that the plasma concentration and bioavailability of hCG was much higher after the IM injections. The study also found that bioavailability in the obese women was lower when compared to the non-obese. **http://tinyurl.com/hcgIM**

More references that IM is faster absorption: **http://tinyurl.com/hcgIM2** and **http://tinyurl.com/hcgIM3**

However, this study found exactly the opposite results: **http://tinyurl.com/hcgSC** The administration methods of this study are not clearly outlined and one study questioned whether in fact the IM might have actually also been SC because the delivery to the muscle was not confirmed by ultrasound.

And this one says that the absorption is the same: **http://tinyurl.com/hcgIMSC**

This one with men and hCG states that SC is slower absorption than IM, but that the half-life is longer, and the steroidogenesis (production of steroids by living organisms) responses make them equally effective for that purpose: **http://tinyurl.com/hcgIMSCBio**

Another pharmacokinetic study comparing SC and IM injections in general found that absorption is dependent on the blood flow to the injection site. More blood flow means more and faster absorption. In general, muscle contains more blood vessels than subcutaneous fat, making IM better and faster absorption. **http://tinyurl.com/hcgIMSCPKCom**

To summarize, the following two tables compare the administration methods:

Comparison of Injection Methods			
Abbreviation	SC or SQ	IM	IV
Full Name	SubCutaneous	IntraMuscular	IntraVenous*
Absorption rate	slow	faster	nearly immediate
Gauge of Needles	29 to 33 gauge	25 to 30 gauge	N/A
Usual Length of Needles	1/2 inch	1 inch or 1 ¼ inch	N/A

*hCG shots are NOT given intravenously.

Subcutaneous Advantages	Intramuscular Advantages
Greater area for target injection sites.	Can give greater volume of drug product (2 to 5 ml as compared to 1 ml for SC).
Fewer landmarks required for targeting injection sites.	Drugs irritating to SC tissue may be given IM.
Shorter needles can be used (3/8 to 5/8 inch compared to 1 to 2 inches for IM).	
Readily self-administered.	
Muscle mass not an issue.	
Less discomfort and inconvenience for patients with neurological disease or limited mobility.	
Better safety profile.	

Is there any way to avoid injections, but still be using real hCG?

One alternative is a mixture that is taken sublingually (under the tongue), because blood vessels are very close to the surface there. Therefore, they are able to absorb anything put under the tongue. For example, sublingual Vitamin B-12 is on drugstore counters. Most mixtures are designed to be held under the tongue for 30 to 45 seconds and then swallowed. You can do the same for the hCG. This method of taking remedies is not new, although many drugs are just being formulated this way. Homeopathic tinctures have been given sublingually for centuries.

Releana is a sublingual patent-pending **http://tinyurl.com/Releana** form of real prescription hCG available to purchase from medical doctors associated with **http://www.releana.com**. A bottle containing a one-month supply costs $250 at the time of publication, including a month of potassium pills. The company also has a list of doctors that make it available to their patients. Releana uses Dr. Simeons' food list except for the omission of the orange, grissini, and melba toast, and the inclusion of broccoli, cauliflower, and 2 diet sodas a day. Patients reportedly have taken Releana for months without any problems. Releana is reported to have a 60-day expiration from the time of purchase (not the time of opening), but must be kept cold. Therefore, it is either shipped overnight in insulated cooled containers or is shipped unmixed and only mixed at the point of destination on the beginning day of the protocol.

Dr. Daniel Belluscio, (**http://hcgobesity.org** and **http://oralhcg.com**), also has developed an hCG sublingual formula and the Releana patent filing cites his studies, indicating that he developed a formula first. One of my diet group members lives in Argentina and is his patient.

Interestingly, Dr B now has two new patents filed on hCG, one for an "oral" (sublingual) administration method and one for using it to treat mood disorders and alcoholism: **http://tinyurl.com/BPatent**
http://tinyurl.com/BPatent2

If you are needle-phobic, members of my diet support group have tested different sublingual recipes and have found even the simplest method to be effective, although the time that the potency of various mixtures remains effective seems to vary. For those who would like to make their own sublingual solution, there are simple ways to "mix your own".

Sublingual hCG

One of the clinic websites states that there is no oral hCG. I guess that strictly speaking, that is correct. hCG cannot be absorbed into the bloodstream orally through the digestive tract. However, it

CAN be absorbed into the bloodstream by holding it under the tongue, which is called sublingual absorption. There IS effective sublingual hCG, with not one, but two patents having been filed now. When using sublingual, the digestive tract is bypassed altogether: **http://tinyurl.com/subling**. Some have been experimenting with homemade formulas of sublingual hCG with great success.

I see a legitimate basis for the sublingual method in Pounds and Inches, in fact. Dr. S discussed alternate methods for absorbing hCG other than using injections. He discussed that when treating the 'fat boys' that it could be absorbed rectally just as well as through injections and was just as effective when administered in that way because the rectal blood vessels are close to the surface.

Administering drugs through sublingual delivery is a method with proven success because the blood vessel-rich mucous membranes in the mouth allow them to be absorbed directly into the bloodstream. By increasing the dosage level, any reduction of absorption caused by such factors as too little time held under the tongue or having eaten or drunk something too close to the time that the dose was taken can be minimized. Also, theoretically, because it is absorbed into the bloodstream instead of IM or SQ, it breaks down much quicker than the other two methods and needs to be taken twice a day to remain in circulation. A person would need to use more hCG and therefore spend more money than someone using one of the injection methods, but that is an expense that many are willing to bear in order to reap the benefits of the convenience and ease of sublingual administration. Increasing the IM dose by 30% results in a dose of 166 IU per day. An increase of 100% is a dose of 250 IU per day. Going to the commercially available sublingual product level is an increase of about 267% for a dose of 333 IU per day. Although this dose seems high enough to induce immunity sooner, the Releana dosage is 333 IU per day with claims of no immunity resulting from this dose.

What dosage of hCG should I take?

It is a personal decision. On page 41, Dr. Simeons states that, "Though a pregnant woman can produce as much as one million units per day, we find that the injection of only 125 units per day is ample to reduce weight at the rate of roughly one pound per day, even in a colossus weighing 400 pounds, when associated with a 500-Calorie diet." In fact he writes on page 84 that "125 I.U. … is the standard dose for all cases and which should never be exceeded." On page 49 he states, "If the daily dose of HCG is raised to 200 or more units daily its action often appears to be reversed, possibly because larger doses evoke diencephalic counter-regulations." KT recommends 175 IU or 200 IU daily because of the assumption that general deterioration of food quality and system-wide toxins require a higher dose to produce the same result in the modern age. The results in my support group haven't necessarily supported that theory. People have been successful at dosages ranging from 125 IU to 250 IU. Variation in dosage does sometimes change people's level of hunger, however. Some of the largest did fine on 150 IU. There are some people who have reported starting at very high doses and then lowering it and getting better results. With hCG, more isn't necessarily better. Sublingual hCG is thought to require a dosage of 250-333 IU and that amount is divided into two doses 12 hours apart because less is absorbed using that method of administration, with a possibility of being broken down faster as well. Subcutaneous injections are usually given in a slightly larger dose because less is absorbed because of less blood flow and also at a slower rate than intramuscular. Some hCG clinics use 250 IU subcutaneously, but some of their patients in my support group have gotten better results by lowering that dose to 200 or 175 IU.

Where can I find suppliers of hCG?

Clinics or private physicians can prescribe it. It is available without prescription in some countries, such as Mexico. Overseas internet pharmacies will provide it by mail-order. This book includes a list of clinics and suppliers, as well as data about them.

hCG Suppliers

The alternatives for obtaining hCG are to get it from a doctor or clinic, take a trip to Mexico or another country in which a prescription is not required at a pharmacy, or to order it from overseas and do it yourself.

When purchased out of the country, it has to go through customs. Some make it through; some don't. Hypothetically speaking, of course, a person would want to be sure to purchase from a place that in the event of a confiscated shipment will re-send the product at no additional charge.

Scam Prevention

If you are concerned about providing your credit card information to buy hCG online, you can go to any CVS pharmacy or Wal-Mart and buy a prepaid Visa to use online. It's $5 or so, for a $100 prepaid VISA card. You use it exactly like a normal credit card except that after you've charged all $100 on it, you throw it away.

From Jeni, the editor of **www.hcgdietinfo.com**:
"hcgdietinfo.com's hCG Provider Directory has recently received a growing number of requests from websites AND individuals (mostly from South America) claiming to sell HCG via mail order, requiring bank or Western Union wire transfers for payment.

Before you order hCG or supplies from abroad, contact your credit card company ahead of time and make sure you will be covered in the event the company does not follow through. A new ring of fraudulent hCG prescription websites have sprung up, requesting Western Union payments or bank wire transfers as payment with no intention of shipping orders. Using PayPal, MasterCard, or Visa protects you from this sort of scam, but DO NOT SEND MONEY TO INTERNATIONAL PHARMACIES VIA WIRE TRANSFER - EVER!"

Ordering Information

hCG is sold under many brand names and is provided by pharmaceutical companies such as Schering, Serono, Squib, Ferring, Organon, Parke-Davis, Wyeth Ayerst, Steris, Fujisawa, and others. Brands of hCG from India would be Corion or Profasi made by Serono. Pregnyl, made by Organon is ordered from Europe/Greece. Lepori, made by Farma-Lepori, is from Spain. IBSA Choriomon is NOT made in Mexico, but is available at pharmacies there. It is from Switzerland.

Here is a handy table listing most of the names for hCG:

Brand Name	IU	Manufacturer
APL (US, SA)	5000, 10000 or 20000 IU	Wyeth-Ayerst
Abraxis		Abraxis Pharmaceutical Products (APP)
Antuitrin S		Parke-Davis
Biogonadyl (PL)	500 or 2000 IU	Biomed
Chorionic Gonadotropin		Steris or Fujisawa
Choragon (G)	1500 or 5000 IU	Ferring Pharmaceuticals
Chorex-5; Chorex-10;Chorex (US)	5000 or 10000 IU	Hyrex
Chorigon		
Choriolife		Life Medicare
Choriolutin (G)		
Choriomon	5000 IU	IBSA, Switzerland
Choron 10 (US)	1000 or 10000 IU	Forest
Chorvlon (A)		
Corgonject		

Brand Name	IU	Manufacturer
Corion		Win Medicare
Dinaron		
Ekluton (G)		
Endocorion		
Fertigyn		Sun Pharmaceuticals (Inca Division)
Follutein		Squib
G. Chor. "Endo" (FR)	500, 1500 or 5000 IU	Organon
Gestyl (BG)	1000 IU	Organon
Glukor (US)		
Gonacor		
Gonadatrophon (GB)	500,1000 or 500 IU	Paines & Byrne
Gonadotraphon LH (I)	125, 250, 1000, 2000 or 5000 IU	Amsa
Gonadotropyl-C (MX/FR)	5000 IU	Roussel
Gonakor (MX)	2500 IU	Sanfer
Gonic (US)	1000 IU	Roberts
Gonotrop-C		Modi-Mundipharma
Harvatropin (US)		
HCG (US)	5000 or 10000 IU	Pharmed
HCG (US)	5000 or 10000 IU	Steris
HCG Lepori (ES)	500, 1000 or 2500 IU	Lepori
Hucog		Bharat Serum & Vaccines
LG IVF - C		LG Life Sciences
Life		Solvay Pharma
Neogonadil Bruco		
Novarel®		Ferring Pharmaceuticals
Ovidac		Zydus Cadila
Ovidrel		Serono
Ovogest (G)		
Ovo-Gonadon (G)		
Ovutrig - HP		VHB Life Sciences
Physex (DK,NO)	1500 or 3000 IU	Leo
Physex Leo (ES)	500,1500 or 5000 IU	Leo
Praedyn (CZ)	1500 or 3000 IU	Leciva
Predalon (G)	500 or 5000 IU	Organon
Pregnesin (G,CZ)	250, 500, 1000, 2500 or 5000 IU	Serono
Pregnyl		Organon India (Infar)
Pregnyl (A,B,CH,GB,BG,GR,I, NL,PL,S,FI,YU,CZ,NO,HU)	5000 IU	Organon
Pregnyl (BG)	100 IU	Organon
Pregnyl (US)	10000 IU	Organon
Primogonyl (CH,G,CZ)	250 or 500 IU	Schering
Primogonyl (G,CH,YU,CZ)	/vials IU	Schering
Profasi (A,B,CH,DK,HU,GB, GR,S,FR,NL,NO,MX)	2000 or 5000 IU	Serono Serum International
Profasi (CH,B,MX,S,FI,GB,NO,NL)	10000 IU	Serono
Profasi (CH,GB,MX,HU,FR)	500 IU	Serono
Profasi (FR)	1500 IU	Serono
Profasi (HU,NL,MX)	1000 IU	Serono
Provigil hCG h		Maneesh Pharmaceuticals
Pubergen		Uni - Sankyo
Rochoric (US)		
ZY - HCG		Zydus Cadila (Biogen Division)

Ordering information for hCG

hCG for a 23-day round with dosage of 125 to 200 IU: 3 1500 to 2000 IU ampoules/vials OR the equivalent in other IU amounts.

hCG for a 43-day round with dosage of 125 to 200 IU: 2 5000 IU ampoules/vials if you are not going to mix more frequently to have fresher hCG OR 6 1500 IU ampoules/vials OR the equivalent in other IU amounts.

Ordering information for IM injection supplies

First, let's talk about your solvent for the hCG. Different formulations of hCG freeze-dried powder are shipped with an appropriate solvent/diluent, which is specific to the excipients in the hCG, to make it the right ph, salts, and so on, to last the longest and not damage the hCG molecule. Some are mixed with bacteriostatic water with 0.9% (less than 1%) benzyl alcohol. Some use bacteriostatic water with 0.56% sodium chloride and 0.9% (less than 1%) benzyl alcohol. Some use 0.9% sodium chloride alone, but those do say to use it immediately and do not claim any stability after mixing. The jury is out as to whether we should be using those formulations for weight reduction, because we use them over a longer period of time, and there is no bacteriostatic agent to prevent bacteria growth.

For our purposes, we need more of the liquid than is typically provided, because we inject smaller doses than for fertility purposes and inject for days at a time, so it needs to last longer. The extra diluent must be purchased separately and must match the original. Some hCG states that it is stable (biologically active undamaged molecule) for 30 days refrigerated, but others state 60 days refrigerated, which must be verified by a biological assay in order to be claimed on the package insert. The formulations and the stability that is claimed correlate.

You may omit the extra needles in the orders listed below, if you wish. Because the needle will be dulled by the rubber stopper on the vial when you withdraw the hCG, many prefer to have extras so they can change to a new needle before injecting.

For 5000 IU ampoules:
- o   1 box (100) of 25g-30g x 1" 3cc luer lock syringe and needle combo (The larger the needle gauge, the smaller the needle size). A smaller needle means less pain (25g-30g seems to be what most are going with).
- o   50-100 extra luer lock 25g–30g x 1" needles
- o   2 30cc sterile vials (amber preferred, but clear will do)
- o   2 30cc syringes
- o   2 30cc vials of appropriate solvent

For 1500 IU ampoules:
- o   1 box (100) of 25g-30g x 1" 3cc luer lock syringe and needle combo (The larger the needle gauge, the smaller the needle size). A smaller needle means less pain (25g-30g seems to be what most are going with).
- o   50-100 extra luer lock 25g–30g x 1" needles
- o   6 10cc sterile vials (amber preferred, but clear will do)
- o   6 10cc syringes
- o   2 30cc vials of appropriate solvent

Ordering information for SC injection supplies

For 5000 IU ampoules:
- o 1 box (100) of 29g-33g x ½" 1cc luer lock syringe and needle combo (The larger the needle gauge, the smaller the needle size). A smaller needle means less pain (29g-33g seems to be what most are going with).
- o 50-100 extra luer lock 29g-33g x ½" needles
- o 2 10cc sterile vials (amber preferred, but clear will do)
- o 2 10cc syringes
- o 2 30cc vials of appropriate solvent

For 1500 IU ampoules:
- o 1 box (100) of 29g-33g x ½" 1cc luer lock syringe and needle combo (The larger the needle gauge, the smaller the needle size). A smaller needle means less pain (29g-33g seems to be what most are going with).
- o 50-100 extra luer lock 29g-33g x ½" needles
- o 6 10cc sterile vials (amber preferred, but clear will do)
- o 6 10cc syringes
- o 2 30cc vials of appropriate solvent

The supplies above will provide you with enough materials to do one 43-day round. You can order less for a 23-day round.

For two 43-day rounds you will need to order:
- o You should order the same amount of syringe/needle combos (100)
- o 100 extra needles (instead of 50)
- o Then double the amount of 10cc or 30ccc syringes
- o Double the amount of sterile vials
- o Double the amount of 30cc vials of appropriate solvent

Ordering information for sublingual supplies

You will need one syringe with a needle, in order to be able to mix your hCG powder initially. You can use any small bottle for storing your sublingual mix, but an amber or cobalt blue glass bottle is recommended, as exposure to sunlight, and so on, can be damaging to the efficacy of formulations. The dark color of the bottle protects the ingredients from damage from light exposure. For accurate dosing, you can order 1cc Tuberculin Syringes & Needles - 25 ga x 5/8" needle (a syringe you will use without the needle, but with accurate markings on the sides) **http://tinyurl.com/subsyr**. You open the bottle, dip the syringe in, pull up to the 0.25 ml line, and squirt under the tongue. Hold there as long as you can and then swallow. Rubber-topped (squeeze bulb) plastic tubes with ml markings found in the baby section can be substituted for a syringe. I like the syringe better for dosing, but something from the baby section can be substituted. Remember ml and cc are the same.

Personally, I prefer using amber or cobalt bottles with dropper tops built in. Here are sources:
http://tinyurl.com/amberbottle
http://tinyurl.com/amberbottle2
http://tinyurl.com/CobaltDropperBottle

To get accurate measurements using the amber bottle dropper top, pull the plain dropper out of the top and replace it with one marked in tenths of a ml, easily obtained from Walgreen's or another drugstore, either online or locally: **http://tinyurl.com/calidropper2 http://tinyurl.com/calidropper**

Many sublingual recipes use such ingredients as some form of drinking alcohol (not recommended as optimal), sublingual Vitamin B-12, or appropriate solvent. Other sublingual liquid vitamins and minerals might work as vehicles as well. Here are a few:

P.L. Chromium Picolinate Sublingual **http://tinyurl.com/SubCP**
B-Complex Sublingual Liquid with B-12 **http://tinyurl.com/SubB12**
American Biologics Taurine Plus **http://tinyurl.com/SubTaurine**
Co Q-10 200 Sublingual by Vitol 2 Oz **http://tinyurl.com/SubCoQ10**
P.L. Zinc Sublingual 2 Oz **http://tinyurl.com/SubZinc**
Vitol Creatine Monohydrate Sublingual 4 Oz **http://tinyurl.com/SubCreatine**

Sources of hCG List

Sources of hCG	Description	Cost	Website / Payment Accepted	Comments
Recommended Top Choice Pharmacy Escrow	5 x 1000 IU 1 x 5000 IU 3 x 5000 IU 3 x 2000 IU	$60.99 $25.99 $72.99 $41.99 $30.00 s&h	http://tinyurl.com/hcglink Visa/Amex/DinersClub Excellent Customer Care 1-877-888-3562 Toll-Free Online Chat Discreet Packaging Email Confirmations And what could be the most important: *Guaranteed Reshipment If Confiscated*	Use Coupon Code 96304 for a Free Gift! 10% off if doubling an order, so put half of what you want in your cart, then double it at the end to get a discount. 3% discount ordering with a check from your bank, but could delay shipment. They do NOT refund, but if it is confiscated, you get notified, and then you contact the company and tell them you don't have it, and they reship it. Contact them and tell them when it has been over a month, and they will give you a $10 coupon and check on your order for you. Delivery: 8 to 21 days.
All Drugs Online	3 x 5000 IU	$69 $10 s&h	http://tinyurl.com/hcglink2 http://tinyurl.com/hcglink3 Visa	$100 minimum order Use the second link to order less than $100. Delivery: 2 to 4 weeks.
Anabolic Pharmacy	1 x 2000 IU 10 x 2000 IU 1 x 5000 IU	$23.04 $195.84 $33.12 $18 s&h	http://tinyurl.com/hcglink4 Visa/MasterCard/Amex	Delivery: 12 days Does NOT reship if confiscated
Best Discounted Pharmacy	1 x 2000 IU 10 x 2000 IU 1 x 5000 IU	$6.00 $55.00 $9.00 $20 s&h	http://tinyurl.com/hcglink5	Delivery: 2 to 4 weeks

Sources of hCG	Description	Cost	Website / Payment Accepted	Comments
Cheap Anabolic	3 x 5000 IU	$45 $15 s&h	http://tinyurl.com/hcglink6 Visa/Amex/DinersClub	$100 minimum order Delivery: 8 to 15 days
Eurobolic	1 x 1500 IU 1 x 5000 IU	$28.00 $40.60 $20 s&h	http://tinyurl.com/hcglink7 Western Union Money Transfer, Direct Bank Transfer, and MoneyGram	Delivery: 8 to 15 days
HCG Mail hCG in 175 IU doses, syringes and needles	1 (23-day) kit 2 kits 3 kits 4 kits 5 kits	$155 $295 $435 $560 $680 $15 s&h	http://tinyurl.com/hcglink8 Bank Transfer or Cashier's Check No phone number provided, Email contact only	Delivery: 10 working days. Sends the package by registered mail.
Reliable Rx	1 x 2000 IU 1 x 5000 IU	$11.79 $17.03 $20 s&h	http://tinyurl.com/hcglink9	Delivery: 10 working days.
Sport Pharma	1 x 1500 IU 1 x 2000 IU 1 x 5000 IU	$20.02 $21.45 $27.17 $20 s&h	http://tinyurl.com/hcglink10 Visa/MasterCard/Western Union	Delivery: 8 to 18 days. Hands your order off to a drop-shipper and therefore canNOT verify whether the order was shipped or give tracking information.
Sustanon Deca	1 x 1500 IU 1 x 5000 IU	$25.74 $36.58 $20 s&h	http://tinyurl.com/hcglink11 Western Union Money Transfer, Direct Bank Transfer, and MoneyGram	Delivery: 10 to 12 days.
United Pharmacy	1 x 1500 IU 1 x 5000 IU	$24.94 $32.28 $22 s&h	http://tinyurl.com/hcglink12 Western Union Money Transfer and MoneyGram	Delivery: 6 to 20 days.

List of Sources of Injection Supplies

Suppliers of Injection Supplies	Description	Cost	Website Address / Forms of Payment Accepted	Comments
HCG Supplies (does not sell hCG) **Recommended Top Choice Especially for Beginners**	hCG-specific Kits with: syringes, needles, alcohol pads, vials, larger syringes for mixing.	Varies by kit. Priority Mail is FREE	**http://tinyurl.com/hcgsupplies** Amex/Visa/MasterCard	Most convenient way to get started. Fast delivery. Most experienced company. Great customer service, very knowledgeable. Free downloadable instructions for dosages and mixing.
AndroUSA	Needles, syringes, vials,	Varies	http://tinyurl.com/supplies1	Fast delivery. Great customer service,

Suppliers of Injection Supplies	Description	Cost	Website Address / Forms of Payment Accepted	Comments
	bacteriostatic water	$9.59 s&h	Amex/Discover/Visa/ MasterCard	very knowledgeable.
GPZ (Got Pinz)	Injection supplies	Varies	http://tinyurl.com/supplies2 Amex/Discover/Visa/ MasterCard	Fast delivery.
Research Supply	Syringes, needles, vials, bacteriostatic water	Varies	http://tinyurl.com/supplies3 Amex/Discover/Visa/ MasterCard/Western Union	Fast delivery. E-mail notification of shipment/tracking.
HCG Coach Kits	Sublingual or injection kits Coaching	Varies by kit	http://tinyurl.com/supplies4	Fast delivery. Great customer service, very knowledgeable.

How can you be sure that what you order online is really hCG?

hCG is a generic commodity pharmaceutical produced in plants all over the world and widely available everywhere, in many countries without a prescription. It's also not very expensive compared to most other pharmaceuticals, especially the patented ones. At the end of the day, if someone's being a pirate, they'd be wasting their time selling fake hCG – faking other more expensive drugs would be much more profitable. Also remember that hCG is a sideline for some of these online pharmacies - their primary business is selling illegal steroids to American bodybuilders. Within that community, if any of them developed a reputation for selling fake products, they'd be out of business. It's just not worth it. Finally, not one of my support group members has said that what they got wasn't hCG - we're talking hundreds of active customers of these pharmacies, all of whom released weight when using the hCG as Simeons prescribed. The only complaints about ineffective hCG came from one person who was using hCG that had expired over a year ago, and several people whose hCG lost potency after sitting in the refrigerator for a few weeks. You can test your hCG solution by putting some drops of it on a pregnancy test to see if it is active, but it does not tell you HOW active it still is, only that it is real hCG and that it is active enough to register on the test.

Is this substance illegal like steroids?

hCG is not illegal and is not a federally-controlled substance, but the FDA has not approved it for use for weight reduction. It is approved for infertility treatment and a rare disease in young boys. It is not illegal for doctors to prescribe it for what is called an off-label use. Doctors have that option at their discretion, although HMO doctors are unlikely to prescribe anything for off-label use due to the restrictions placed on them by most HMOs. There are some clinics that will send you injections through the mail as well. Many have reported that they have ordered, mixed, and done all injections or sublingual dosing based on the information offered in this book.
Please note that this drug is NOT a human growth hormone that could cause the disease acromegaly if overdosing takes place. That hormone is hGH, _not_ hCG. These two substances are completely different, but nonetheless are often confused for some reason.

What are the legal issues surrounding this diet?

I am not a lawyer and this is not legal advice, nor a substitute for it. Consult a legal professional for definitive answers to legal matters. hCG is a prescription drug in the United States. Although it can be obtained from other countries or overseas without one, obtaining it legally in the US requires that you go to a physician and get a prescription. And while hCG is approved for several uses (for instance, infertility), the FDA has not approved it for the uses outlined in this book. I should also note that it is legal for a doctor to prescribe any non-scheduled drug for any condition for which he or she feels it would be beneficial. hCG is not a federally scheduled or controlled substance, and falls into this category; a physician could prescribe it for the uses described in this book, although they are not FDA approved uses.

According to Rick Collins of **www.steroidlaw.com**, *Human chorionic gonadotropin* (hCG) is mistakenly classified as an "anabolic steroid" and a controlled substance (illegal distribution is a felony) in the following states: California, Colorado, Connecticut, Idaho, Indiana, Louisiana, Nevada, New York, North Carolina, Pennsylvania and Rhode Island, although it is not listed as a federally controlled substance. This is because it is used by steroid-using bodybuilders in doses much higher than used for this diet to restart their natural testosterone production again after steroid use.

This book is for informational, educational, review, and entertainment purposes only and does not advocate or promote any illegal activity.

In the late 1980s, the FDA put a new policy into place which allowed US consumers to import up to a 90-day supply of prescription drugs for personal use (i.e. not for resale). This policy was designed to allow AIDS patients and others who suffered from chronic illnesses to import drugs which had not yet undergone FDA approval. However, with the emergence of the Internet, many companies began to offer the US consumers less expensive prescriptions from abroad. The FDA then asserted that the policy only applied to non-FDA approved drugs (which protects US pharmaceutical manufacturers from foreign competition and keeps prices artificially high). The US Congress responded by authoring a plethora of bills stating that the FDA should not prohibit the importation of prescription drugs from abroad as long as such drugs are for personal use (i.e. in no larger than 90-day quantities). While the official FDA policy has not yet changed, the agency has not interfered with importation for personal use as long as the purchaser has a prescription for the drugs being imported. In fact, some local and state governments in the US have begun to buy prescription drugs for their public employees from abroad in order to cut costs, and many more have stated their intentions to begin doing so **http://tinyurl.com/CanadaDrugs**. Illinois created a website that allows its residents to import prescription drugs from abroad. Wisconsin, Kansas, Vermont and Missouri have now joined the site. (Other Recent Developments – **http://tinyurl.com/RICanada, http://tinyurl.com/MNCanada, http://tinyurl.com/WACanada, http://tinyurl.com/ILCanada,** and **http://tinyurl.com/MOCanada**.) Importing prescriptions has become a very hot topic in the last few years, receiving a lot of attention in the presidential primary debates, a feature story on 60 Minutes (**http://tinyurl.com/ArtificiallyHigh**) and other major news programs, and lobbying campaigns for senior advocacy groups such as AARP. The debate still rages. For further information on current legislation and the legalities of importing prescription drugs for personal use, see these links:

Congressional Legislation:
Amendment to Allow for Importation of Prescription Drugs **http://tinyurl.com/PropAmend**
Affordable Medicine Safety and Access Act **http://tinyurl.com/PropAmend2**
Preserving Access to Safe, Affordable Canadian Medicines Act **http://tinyurl.com/PropAmend3**
Importation of Prescription Drug Bill #H.R.1 **http://tinyurl.com/PropAmend4**
Prescription Drug Parity for Americans Act **http://tinyurl.com/PropAmend5**
Save Our Seniors Act **http://tinyurl.com/PropAmend6**

FDA Statement:

50

FDA, "Information on Importation of Drugs," Marvin A. Blumberg, Division of Import Operations and Policy, Office of Regulatory Affairs, FDA, HFC-170, April 3, 1998, at **http://tinyurl.com/FDAPID**
FDA, "Coverage of Personal Importations," *Regulatory Procedures Manual*, Office of Regulatory Affairs, FDA, January 11, 2003, at **http://tinyurl.com/FDAREGMAN**

Hypothetically, if a person ordered a personal supply of hCG from an overseas or internet pharmacy, my understanding is that customs can confiscate it and, if so, the person would receive a letter notifying them that it had been detained by customs. If that person had a prescription, that person might claim it. However, without a prescription, a person would NOT want to claim it, as there would be no proof that they ordered it unless the person did try to claim it. Without any proof, it seems unlikely that anyone would be charged with anything. Hopefully this hypothetical person would have ordered from one of the companies that will reship the order if confiscated by customs.

According to drugs.about.com, "October, 2006 President Bush signed the Department of Homeland Security Appropriations Act, which included a clause prohibiting US Customs and Border Protection from seizing personal prescription drug supplies (up to a 90-day supply) from individuals bringing drugs across the Canada-US border into the US. On the same day, the Department also announced that it would stop seizing mail-ordered prescription drugs at the Canada-US border on their way into the US. These conciliations were a response to a year of protests by individuals, state governments, and congressmen about the government's crackdown on drug importation from Canada, which resulted in many individuals unexpectedly having their medications confiscated.

Both practices remain illegal, however the Department of Homeland Security has made it clear that it does not intend to enforce the laws that apply. This was seen as a sign that full-fledged legalization of prescription drug imports is just around the corner. Opponents of legalization of importation include drug companies (who have an obvious conflict of interest) as well as many congressmen who argue that the closed regulatory system governing drug production and consumption in the US is critical for the protection of US residents. Most recently, May 7, 2007 a bill that would legalize personal-use drug importation was killed in the Senate." **http://tinyurl.com/ImportLaw**

According to the USPS, these are the guidelines for sending medicine through the mail:

"Many medications are not mailable through the mail by individuals. If you are at all unsure as to whether or not the medicine you have is mailable, you should contact your local Post Office for further assistance.

All prescription, nonprescription, and patent medicines and related items, including solicited and unsolicited samples of such items, that are not considered to be controlled substances, are permitted to be mailed as follows:
   o For prescription medicines containing a nonnarcotic drug(s), the mailer must be a registered practitioner or dispenser mailing to the ultimate user.
   o Effective February 2, 2006, consumers may mail prescription drugs if/when returning them to drug manufacturers or their agents, pharmacies, and other authorized dispensers and only when the authorized entity provides the consumer with a mailing container bearing a merchandise return service permit indicia.
   o For nonprescription medicines, the mailer must meet all applicable federal, state, or local laws that may apply."

Step 15 – *Plan your program by deciding your schedule for Phases and rounds.*

Plan your program by deciding your schedule for Phases and rounds, considering holidays, vacations, and special events.

What do I do while I am waiting to receive my hCG?

This is a good time to continue your research and study of the protocol so that you will be ready to begin when you have all the materials required. You can also read the labels on all of the processed food items in your pantry and refrigerator, to eliminate any with obesity-promoting additives such as MSG, high fructose corn syrup, and so forth, since you won't want to eat these foods after you have released weight, in order to avoid regaining. Many people begin Phase 1 with some natural herb cleanses and colonics. Consider using this time to plan out a week or two of menus for Phase 2.

Step 16 – *If necessary, buy scales for weighing yourself and your food.*

Do I have to get a postal scale as Dr. Simeons states?

No, food scales are now electronic and accurate enough to use. The spring-loaded food scales used in his day were not accurate. I got the Salter Digital Scale Model #1008 from Bed Bath & Beyond, which can switch back and forth between grams and ounces. There is also one that tells you all the nutritional information about whatever food you are weighing, which is really cool, but it is more expensive at $100. I bought the $50 model using the 20% off coupon.

The Kitrics Digital Nutrition Scale **http://tinyurl.com/DigitalFoodScale** not only weighs in grams and ounces but also has a food list so you can punch in a code for the type of food you're weighing and it will give you all kinds of nutritional info like calories, fat, sodium.

Phase 1

Step 17 – *Become educated about Cleanses for Phase 1.*

Candida

I'm craving sweets. What can I do?

Kevin Trudeau writes about this problem in his books. Sugar and carbohydrate cravings are caused by an overgrowth of Candida yeast fungi. Did you do a Candida cleanse in Phase 1? You can do some free home testing for Candida overgrowth with an easy test found at: **http://tinyurl.com/SpitTest**. It's simple, fast, and slightly disgusting.

An overgrowth of Candida yeast fungi can only occur if the body is out of balance, having a diminished microflora. Microflora is the good bacteria that lives in your digestive tract, from your stomach to your anus. Our diets, before the chemical revolution, were rich in good bacteria. When we ate an apple, cabbage, drank raw unpasteurized milk, etc., we were consuming loads of good bacteria, as nature intended. Most people are unaware that good bacteria is supposed to be in our diets! Herbicides, pesticides, pasteurization, radiating food, and other farming practices have greatly diminished the amount of bacteria that is available in our diets. A healthy digestive tract has 5 to 7 pounds of good bacteria. These colonies of good bacteria have many functions, including synthesizing one vitamin into another, cleaning the colon lining, eradicating parasites, among other functions. For instance, Vitamin

B-12 is not readily available in the diet and is easily damaged by stomach acids when consumed. Vitamin B-6 is rich in our diets, and one of the functions of microflora is to transform B-6 into B-12. Now, if a person does not have a healthy microflora, they are likely to experience some of the deficiency symptoms of B-12, which include a tightness around the chest, depression, fatigue, a feeling of heaviness, among other things, to varying degrees.

There are a couple of supplements that will help to lower the Candida yeast fungi population; although, the only real way to make sure that the Candida does not overgrow again is to provide the body with sufficient amounts of good bacteria to renourish the microflora. Such things as antibiotics, chlorine, steroids, stress, chemotherapy, excess sugar consumption, and medications are some of the most common causes for an overgrowth of Candida yeast fungi, because Candida is a natural inhabitant, but it is not natural to have large colonies of Candida. Candida can overgrow if the microflora is compromised, and Candida always wrecks havoc on good health.

The challenge is to find the right kind of supplement to address an overgrowth of Candida. You see, our federal government did some testing on nuclear bombs and intentionally exposed various living organisms. The nuclear bombs killed all life, except for Candida yeast fungi and cockroaches. The yeast survived by morphing into another form. This is what occurs when one takes most herbs and it initially appears to 'work'. Typically, within two to three weeks, the cravings and symptoms return.

Two supplements that do not kill the Candida, but instead affect it in another way include Threelac, which actually eats it, and Candida-G, which disables the Candida reproduction mechanism. Remember, these are just tools to lower the Candida population, but do nothing to renourish the microflora and restore the natural balance of the body. FermPlus is necessary for that job to be accomplished. On Phase 2, Candida-G stopped my cravings for sweets and carbs.

Just as hCG will help to reset the hypothalamus, probiotics will help to restore the microflora. Probiotics are nutritional supplements that provide the body with good bacteria. FermPlus is a probiotic that reproduces and colonizes, once consumed. The bacteria in this probiotic superfood is grown in vegetables, is gluten, casein, and milk free, with naturally occurring vitamins, minerals, and amino acids. Some people do well using FermPlus during Phase 1 only, but others find that they improve digestive health more by continuing it during Phases 3 and 4.

My friend Victoria Smith can help you, regardless of how mild or severe your cravings and other Candida-related symptoms are. Through years of research and much trial and error, she has developed a protocol that works every time. She works with people around the world to get rid of an overgrowth of Candida. **www.CandidaExpert.com** is her website. I have worked out a discount for all HCG dieters who buy my e-book, for free shipping on-going. Check out her website and webstore, and upon checkout, use the coupon code CCHCG.

I used to recommend other products, but eventually found out that they provided only temporary results, and those results lasted longer than usual while on the 500 calorie diet, just because of the nature of the food list that we can eat. When we don't eat sugar and carbohydrates, we eliminate the food source for Candida, which is not a bad way to lower the Candida population; however, the most important part of eradicating Candida once and forever is to renourish the microflora. This way, as you move from P2 into P3 and P4, the sugar, carbs, and processed foods just don't taste as good, further supporting your long term weight reduction maintenance by supporting good eating habits. I see in my support group that when people return to their old eating habits as they move into P4, that this is probably why. If they have nurtured a healthy microflora and have gotten their Candida under control,

they don't even want a candy bar, chips, and so forth and in fact, if they do try them, they can 'taste' the added chemicals in these foods because their bodies are in balance.

Heavy Metal

In Phase 2, while we are releasing weight, toxins that were stored in the fat that we are releasing, including heavy metals, are being released into our bodies. Some of the treatments to remove these, for instance heavy metal chelation (such as DMSA or IV pushes) typically pose some problems. Each has its drawbacks and dangers. As an example, they chelate minerals that we need, they stir up sequestered toxins, toxins can redistribute in tissue, making the end result worse than before treatment.

To my knowledge, the only detox product that is okay to take to clean this up during Phase 2 is Natural Cellular Defense (NCD), a liquid zeolite dietary supplement. NCD can absorb the toxins and carry them out of our bodies. It has the ability to help remove environmental toxins such as heavy metals from the body to detoxify the body. It has the ability to support and stabilize a healthy immune system. It has the ability to balance and stabilize a healthy pH level in the body. No minerals that we need are removed. No redistribution occurs. It works 100 per cent of the time. And it works passively, because it does not stimulate the release of any stored toxins. Instead, it moves with blood flow, attracting and binding toxins irreversibly within a cage-like structure to eliminate them from the body.

Think of Zeolite as a combination of a sponge and a magnet that has a negative charge. When it attracts and binds enough positively charged toxins to become net neutral charged, the body simply eliminates the now-toxic zeolite cage. It is 100 per cent natural, non-toxic, and safe for long-term use. In fact, Zeolite is listed as having FDA GRAS status: **http://tinyurl.com/ZeoliteGRAS** under 21 CFR Part 582.2729.

Zeolites are natural volcanic minerals with a unique, complex crystalline structure. Its honeycomb framework of cavities and channels (like cages) works at the cellular level trapping, heavy metals and toxins. In fact, because it is one of the few negatively charged minerals in nature, zeolites act as magnets drawing toxins to it, capturing them in its cage and removing them from the body.

It's important to understand that there are more than 100 different zeolites. As an example, asbestos is a zeolite and causes cancer when inhaled as a fine powder. The zeolite used in the Natural Cellular Defense is naturally-occurring non-fibrous clinoptilolite and is considered to be extremely safe and entirely non-toxic (even when inhaled). A study published in 1993 concluded that "clinoptilolite type zeolite had no carcinogenic activity." (Tatrai E, Ungvary G. Study on carcinogenicity of clinoptilolite type zeolite in Wistar rats. Pol J Occup Med Environ Health. 1993;6(1): 27-34.)

In fact, the type of zeolite [clinoptilolite] used in NCD was utilized after the Chernobyl incident in Russia to remove radioactive strontium and cesium because normal excretion of radioactive compounds has been shown to be up-regulated with zeolite. In three separate studies specifically analyzing the ability of clinoptilolite to aid in the excretion of radioactive cesium particles, the zeolite was found to accelerate the excretion of Cs-137 from sheep's bodies. The whole effect resulted in 15 to 50 times lowering of the equilibrium concentration of the radiocaesium. (Jandl J, Novosad J. [In vivo reduction of radiocesium with modified clinoptilolite in sheep] Vet Med (Praha). 1995 Aug; 40(8): 237-41.)

This paper has information with photos concerning zeolite properties and uses:
http://tinyurl.com/Zeolites (Mumpton, Frederick A. [La roca magica: Uses of natural zeolites in agriculture and industry] Proc Natl Acad Sci U S A. 1999 March 30; 96(7): 3463–3470.)

You can order NCD Zeolite from **http://tinyurl.com/Waiora** at a discount by becoming a distributor.

NCD does help with Candida to some extent, but for a full Candida protocol to eliminate it forever, I suggest working with Victoria, who has graciously given me a discount code for her web store, **www.significanthealing.com/cart**, for free shipping for all of us HCG dieters. The code is CCHCG to use when checking out. There is a coupon on the last page of this book for you to use to get a free 5-minute consultation with Victoria.

Step 18 – Purchase and use cleanses and other Phase I options, if you choose to do so.

Step 19 – Become educated about organic food.

Eating Organic

Dr. Simeons did not tell us to eat organic. You have to remember, he did this in the 50's, 60's, and 70's and in Rome. (At that time, even US food did not have all the toxins that it does today). Even today, the Europeans do not add all the hormones and antibiotics to their livestock and I believe that is one of the reasons why it is North Americans that are so obese and Europeans are not.

I believe that if you continue to ingest all the chemical pesticides, toxins, growth hormones, and antibiotics, you'll gain back everything you released in a couple of years. After detoxing and releasing the weight, I don't want to have to do it all over again. I am encouraged by the increased availability that I see now in organic foods, brought on, no doubt, by consumers demanding it. Regarding the increased costs of eating organic, the average cost increase is 15% - 30% depending on location.

I know that in this day and age it is impossible to eat only organic and there will be times that I will eat non-organic food, such as in restaurants, but why over stress my system on a regular basis? That being said, ultimately, it is your choice.

What does organic mean?

100% organic, that's the best. The next is probably certified organic, then organic and last would be made with organic, which means next to nothing.

How can I tell if produce is organic?

PLU Produce Codes **www.PLUcodes.com**
9=organic; Add a '9' in front of the four digit PLU code. An organically grown standard yellow banana would be '94011'.
8=GE; Add an '8' in front of the four digit PLU code. A genetically engineered standard yellow banana would be '84011'.
http://tinyurl.com/PLUguide

What is a GMO?

A genetically modified organism (GMO) is a plant, animal or microorganism whose genetic code has been altered (subtracted from, or added to either the same species or a different species) in order to give it characteristics that it does not have naturally.

Scientists can now transfer genes between species that otherwise would be incapable of mating, for example, a goat and a spider. This is what we call transgenesis. Little is known about the long-term effects of such manipulations on humans, plants, animals and/or the environment. And while some see GMOs as the way to the future, others believe that scientists have gone too far, tinkering with the essence of life.

What is the difference between "all natural" and "organic"?

All natural refers to no additives and *is based on testimony of the producer*. **Organic** means the product comes from at least 90% organic ingredients, but **100% organic** means 100% of the ingredients are organic. **Certified organic** must come from animals whose parents were certified raised organic and raised from birth on organic land. They must be fed organic crops. The land cannot have been sprayed with pesticides, herbicides, fungicides, or synthetic fertilizers for a minimum of 3 years prior to certification. No animal byproducts may be fed to certified organic animals. No genetically engineered organisms (GMOs) may be used in feed or the animals. The product to be certified must be documented from birth to purchaser for traceability and verification. Antibiotics cannot be used in organic meat.

What is the difference between all the different types of meat?

I did some research on meat and spoke to my butcher. This is the information that I received.

o **Regular beef** is usually kept very contained and fed hormones, antibiotics and supplements as well as grains, and ground-up animal by-products. Most of the animal by-products are from animals that were sick and not fit for human consumption. (Cows are not supposed to eat meat!!) Since the animals are contained, they don't get any exercise and toxins aren't able to be released from their bodies.

o Some animals are given all the hormones, antibiotics, and supplements as well as the grains and animal by-products but allowed time to roam free. In my area this is called **free-range meat**.

o **All natural beef** starts its life as regular beef but is allowed to roam free in the fields and is not given any hormones, antibiotics, or supplements for at least the last few months of its life. It is still fed grains. It's better than regular beef.

o **Organic beef** is never given any hormones, antibiotics, supplements, etc. Neither have their parents. They are never given any feed that is grown with the use of pesticides or chemical fertilizers. (The ground can't have been sprayed for at least 3 years where the feed is grown.) The animals are treated by natural methods if they become ill. If that doesn't work and the farmer needs to use an injection to cure the animal, it is labeled and sold as regular beef. These animals are free to roam their entire life. They are also fed grains.

o **Grass fed only organic beef** is never fed grains. They eat in the fields and are fed hay when weather doesn't permit them to free graze. The proven benefits of eating "Grass-Only Beef" include: less fat, fewer calories, more Omega-3 fatty acids, a healthier ratio of Omega-6 to Omega-3 fatty acids, more Conjugated Linoleic Acid (CLA), more Vitamin E and higher levels of beta-carotene. This is the best meat.

Here is a tip for everyone not eating organic – use Veggie Wash. It is natural, grapefruit oil (which is allowed on the diet – but needless to say you wash it off anyway). It is supposed to remove something like 98% of all pesticides, etc. And while you are at it – tell everyone you know about it – especially those with children as their little bodies are even more sensitive to those chemicals. You can find it in grocery stores, health food stores, Wal-Mart – and online. Citrus Magic Veggie Wash 16 Oz **http://tinyurl.com/VeggieWash**

You also may be getting lots of toxins from what you put on your skin. This article states that we absorb close to **five pounds** of chemicals a year from daily makeup: **http://tinyurl.com/absorbcosmetics**. To assess a particular product's ingredients, you can use **www.cosmeticdatabase.com**, which provides a grading on how harmful that ingredient might be in addition to any studies, side effects, complaints, and list of existing products where you find the ingredient in question.

Step 20 – Determine sources for organic food, if you choose to do so.

How do I find organic foods?
http://www.eatwellguide.org should tell you where there are local places to eat and shop. Also, if you have the time, watch the Meatrix videos. It spoofs the Matrix, but is about farming practices: **http://www.themeatrix.com**. A Texas chiropractor has posted some help with this on his website: **http://tinyurl.com/OrganicSources**. Keep in mind that this list contains all foods, not just those that are allowed while taking hCG injections. When on Phases 1, 3, or 4, those other food listings could be helpful to find organic sources.

While superstores like Wal-Mart, Target, and Kmart are continually expanding their organic foods sections, you will find larger varieties at all-natural grocery stores such as Whole Foods, Alfalfas, Wild Oats, Trader Joe's, and even local farmer's markets. Another option that dieters rarely think of, are international markets. Asian food markets often have extensive organic sections, as do Latin markets. You can also use this handy online resource to locate the purest foods in your area, hormone free meats, organic food etc: **http://tinyurl.com/WPrice**

Step 21 – Begin purchasing and eating organic, if you choose to do so.

Step 22 – Visit www.hcgdietingstore.com to see some products that can be used on the protocol.
Visit **www.hcgdietingstore.com** to see many products that can be used on the protocol.

Step 23 – Change to protocol-compliant personal care products, if you choose to do so.

Dr. Simeons states not to use oils except mineral oil. If I am a massage therapist, nail technician, or cosmetologist and have to apply creams and oils to my clients all day, what can I do?
"...fats, oils, creams and ointments applied to the skin are absorbed and interfere with weight reduction by HCG just as if they had been eaten," according to Simeons. Either use nitrile gloves or a no-oil massage gel such as **www.IncrEdiblEarth.com**, which has only white clay and seaweed as ingredients. Nitrile exam gloves made by McKessen or Kimberly Clark are a little thicker, they don't spin around on your hand, don't breakdown and tear from chemical or oils, and you don't lose the sensitivity that you need. **http://www.dontheglove.com/nitrilegloves/**

What can I do for my dry skin?

I bought a pair of those loofah gloves that take the dry skin off, which you can find in the body care section of most drug stores or variety stores. Just use your regular soap in the shower with the gloves to slough off the dead skin. I've done it for years and it really helps. Most report that their skin is more hydrated and supple while on hCG, but if you must use something, try oil-free moisturizers, such as plain "Aloe Vera" that contains Vitamin E and grapefruit seed extract. My dear friend Shalom puts it into a spray bottle and spritzes lips, face, neck and elbows periodically and upon waking and before bedtime. **http://tinyurl.com/AloeGel** Aubrey Organics 100% Pure Aloe Vera Gel, 4 Oz. Another suggestion is to use Pretty Feet and Hands to remove dry dead skin before spraying the Aloe. You can also try Alba Oil-Free moisturizer **http://tinyurl.com/AlbaOilFree**, or TwinLab Na-PCA Spray **http://tinyurl.com/NaPCASpray**, which many have used without a stall. Nutritive oils that could be absorbed by the skin as "food" are the ones to watch out for. Examples would be olive oil, almond oil, and the like. Oils that are okay are mineral oils and essential oils such as lavender.

Skin Care for Phase 2

One way to continue to moisturize during this time that will NOT affect your hCG is to get a small spray bottle **http://tinyurl.com/FineMister** suitable for misting your body and face. Get a smaller one **http://tinyurl.com/SmallFineMister** to stick in your purse as well. Fill it with purified water and Sea Salt. About 1 tablespoon for a 12 ounce bottle. Shake before spraying. This attracts the moisture from the air to keep your skin and hair moisturized. Also, instead of your regular cleanser switch to Seventh Generation Baby Wipes as a way to cleanse your face and remove make up while maintaining your ph level. This will ensure your skin's protective barrier stays intact.

Oil-free Sunblocks

Coppertone Sunscreen Lotion, Oil Free, SPF15, 8 Oz **http://tinyurl.com/OilFreeSuntan**
Peter Thomas Roth Ultra Lite Oil-Free Sunblock SPF30, 4 Oz **http://tinyurl.com/PeterRoth**
Yes, there is such a thing as organic sunblock: DDF Organic Sun Protection SPF30 4 Oz **http://tinyurl.com/DDFSunS**

Moisturizers

I found an organic spray moisturizer: Twinlab Na-PCA Non Oily Spray 8 Fl Oz **http://tinyurl.com/NaPCASpray2**
Some like this one, but it is not organic and contains some questionable ingredients: Corn Huskers Heavy Duty Oil-Free Hand Lotion 7 Oz **http://tinyurl.com/CHuskers** I used it on my face and it feels soft and absorbed well.

It's Not Easy to be Clean…

Oil-free shampoo: Mastey Shampoo Traite 32 Oz **http://tinyurl.com/Mastey**
or Mastey Volumizing Shampoo Enove 32 Oz **http://tinyurl.com/Mastey2**
Oil-free conditioner:_Mastey Frehair Conditioner 32 Oz **http://tinyurl.com/Mastey3**
or Mastey Frehair Light **http://tinyurl.com/Mastey4**
Deodorant: No aluminum and you only apply it every few days: NOW Foods, Lavilin Underarm Deodorant Cream, **http://tinyurl.com/Lavilin**
Toothpaste: **http://tinyurl.com/TooSoap**

Step 24 – Mentally prepare for Phase 2.

Phase 2

Step 25 – Review the section in the book on the Recipes for the diet plan and food preparation.

The allowed food list is:

BREAKFAST: Tea or coffee in any quantity without sugar. Only one tablespoonful of milk allowed in 24 hours. Saccharin or other sweeteners may be used.

LUNCH:

1. 100 grams of veal, beef, chicken breast, fresh white fish, lobster, crab, or shrimp. All visible fat must be carefully removed before cooking, and the meat must be weighed raw. It must be boiled or grilled without additional fat. Salmon, eel, tuna, herring, dried or pickled fish are not allowed. The chicken breast must be removed raw from the bird.
2. One type of vegetable only to be chosen from the following: spinach, chard, chicory, beet-greens, green salad, tomatoes, celery, fennel, onions, red radishes, cucumbers, asparagus, cabbage.
3. One breadstick (grissino) or one Melba toast.
4. An apple or an orange or a handful of strawberries or one-half grapefruit.

DINNER: The same four choices as lunch.

Is there a cookbook to help with recipes for Phase 2 (hCG injection phase)?

Yes, my friend Tammy created a fantastic one! She has allowed me to use a few recipes in this section. The full cookbook is available at **http://tinyurl.com/hcgcookbook**.

hCG Phase 2 Recipes

Eating this way doesn't have to be boring. Although calorie counts are not listed, most of the main dish recipes are about 140 calories per serving, leaving room for some afternoon snacks.

Any food listed in these recipes should be understood to be organic, to comply with that requirement if you are following it. The only sweetener that is listed is stevia, to comply with that requirement if you are following it. Broth should be nonfat and sugar-free, with NO MSG. Water should be from a pure source. Apple Cider Vinegar should be raw, unfiltered with the "mother". Chicken (breast only allowed) is boneless and skinless. I have tried to avoid any mixing of vegetables, but a very few of the recipes do have more than one, in which case, I have indicated so. Some people have reported no affect on weight reduction.

I use tomatoes as both vegetables and fruit, depending on the recipe, and it has not impaired my weight reduction at all. Your mileage may vary.

T = Tablespoon
t = teaspoon
C = Cup

Don't miss my "Tips" section at the end!

Beverages

Simeons Soda
1 C Brewed Tea of choice
1 to 2 C Ice Cubes
1 Drinking Straw
2 packets Stevia Powder
1 - 1 1/2 C Mineral Water
Brew the tea. Add ice cubes to a large cup. Sprinkle stevia over the ice. Add cooled tea, fill the rest of the cup with mineral water and mix.
10 minutes

Citrus Soda
Juice of 1 Lemon
1 or 2 C Ice
2 packets Stevia Powder
1 Drinking Straw
1 - 1 ½ C Mineral Water
Fill the cup with the amount of ice you desire. Squeeze the juice in the cup. Sprinkle stevia over ice and lemon. Add mineral water and enjoy.

Strawberry Frappe
5 - 6 Strawberries
4 ounces Cold Water
1 C Ice Cubes
1 C Mineral Water
3 teaspoons Stevia

Put all the ingredients in a good blender and mix well. Serve in a tall cup with a straw.
5 minutes

Lemonade
Water
½ Lemon
Stevia
Squeeze half a lemon in a glass of water and add stevia to taste.
5 minutes

P2 hot chocolate can be made by using Chocolate-flavored stevia and hot water.

Instant Yerba Mate: **http://tinyurl.com/YerbaMateInstant**

Yerba Mate Chocolatte: **http://tinyurl.com/YerbaChocolatte**

Celestial Seasonings Chai Tea, Chocolate Caramel Enchantment, **http://tinyurl.com/ChocCara**
Zero calories and zero everything. I added some stevia and it was heavenly.

Herbal Coffee: Teeccino All-Purpose Grind, Hazelnut, Caffeine-Free Herbal Coffee,
http://tinyurl.com/teeccino

Celestial Seasonings Ice Cool Brew Iced Tea, Peach, Tea Bags, **http://tinyurl.com/PeachCool**

Make your own flavored waters

Root Beer – 1 cup sparkling water plus 8 drops SweetLeaf Sweetleaf Stevia Liquid Sweetner Root
Beer 2 oz **http://tinyurl.com/RootBeerStevia**

Chocolate Raspberry – 1 cup water plus 8 drops SweetLeaf Stevia Clear Liquid Chocolate
Raspberry 2 oz **http://tinyurl.com/ChocRasp**

Lemon Drop – 1 cup water plus 7 drops Sweetleaf Stevia Liquid Sweetener Lemon Drop 2 oz
http://tinyurl.com/LemonDropStevia

Grape – 1 cup water plus 7 drops Sweetleaf Stevia Liquid Grape Flavor 2 oz
http://tinyurl.com/GrapeStevia

Orange Julius – 1 cup water plus 7 drops Sweetleaf Stevia Liquid Sweetener Valencia Orange 2 oz
http://tinyurl.com/ValOrange and 2 drops Sweetleaf Stevia Liquid Sweetener Vanilla Creme 2 oz
http://tinyurl.com/VanillaCreme

Chocolate Toffee – 1 cup water plus 7 drops SweetLeaf Clear Liquid Stevia Dark Chocolate 2 oz
http://tinyurl.com/DarkChoco and 3 drops Sweetleaf Liquid Stevia English Toffee 2 oz
http://tinyurl.com/EngToffee

Chocolate Mint – 1 cup water plus 7 drops SweetLeaf Clear Liquid Stevia Dark Chocolate 2 oz
http://tinyurl.com/DarkChoco and 4 drops SweetLeaf Liquid Stevia Peppermint 2 oz
http://tinyurl.com/PeppermintStevia

Chocolate Cinnamon – 1 cup water plus 6 drops SweetLeaf Clear Liquid Stevia Dark Chocolate 2 oz
http://tinyurl.com/DarkChoco and 6 drops Sweetleaf Stevia Liquid Sweetener Cinnamon 2 oz
http://tinyurl.com/CinnamonStevia

These are delicious flavor drops with no sweetener whatsoever that you can use with any sweetener:
http://tinyurl.com/CapellaFlavorDrops I use Creme Brulee flavor in my morning coffee with stevia.

For the Recipes

Bragg Liquid Aminos - 32 oz - Liquid **http://tinyurl.com/Bragg32**
Bragg Liquid Aminos 16 Oz **http://tinyurl.com/Bragg16**
Bragg Liquid Aminos Spray 6 Oz **http://tinyurl.com/Bragg6**

Bragg - Apple Cider Vinegar, gallon, 1 **http://tinyurl.com/ACVGallon**
Bragg - APL CIDR VINGR,OG,RAW - 32 OZ **http://tinyurl.com/ACVQuart**
Bragg - APL CIDR VINGR,OG,RAW - 16 OZ **http://tinyurl.com/ACVPint**

Dressings, Sauces, Salsas, Seasonings, and Marinades

Basic Dressing
3 T Bragg's Amino Acids
Apple Cider Vinegar
1 ½ packet Stevia
¼ t White Pepper
¼ t Cayenne Pepper

Another Basic Dressing
Apple Cider Vinegar
Garlic, minced
Oregano
Basil
Stevia

Dressing for Veggies
Dill Weed
Apple Cider Vinegar
Stevia
Sprinkle fresh dill on any veggie after marinating lightly in Apple Cider Vinegar. If needed, add a little stevia. This really brings out the natural flavor.

Dressing for Cucumbers
Apple Cider Vinegar
Bragg's Amino Acids
Stevia

Strawberry Vinaigrette Dressing *A Tammy Recipe (This is a recipe from my wonderful friend, Tammy. To get more of her great Phase 2 recipes, go to: **http://tinyurl.com/hcgcookbook**.
Strawberries
1-2 tablespoons apple cider vinegar
1 tablespoon lemon juice
Stevia to taste
Dash of salt
Dash of cayenne (optional)
Fresh ground black pepper to taste
Stevia to taste
Combine all ingredients in food processor. Puree until smooth. Pour over fresh arugala or green salad. Garnish with sliced strawberries and freshly ground black pepper. Variation: use as a marinade or sauce. Makes 1 serving (1 fruit)

Umeboshi Plum Paste Dressing
This is a bit of a cheat, since pickled foods are not allowed on Simeons' protocol, but it is nice for a change of pace once in a while. Umeboshi are Japanese salted pickled plums in the macrobiotic section of Whole Foods. They are considered medicine for digestive disorders in old Japanese medicine. You can also get Umeboshi Plum Vinegar. Blend a tiny bit of the paste with quite a bit of water, a dash of Bragg's amino acids, plenty of stevia to taste, and some herbs and spices. You could add some cayenne to this for variety. It's also a great marinade or sauce for protein.

Onion Salad Dressing
1T Chopped Onion
1/4 Lemon, juiced
¼ t Basil
¼ t Oregano
¼ t Cumin
Sea Salt
Freshly Ground Black Pepper

Cocktail Sauce
1 C Sugar-Free Tomato Sauce
1 T Onion Powder
½ T Celery Salt
¼ T Paprika
2 T Fresh Chopped Parsley
1 T Stevia
1 T Worcestershire Sauce
1 T Fresh Lemon Juice
2 T Drained, Prepared Horseradish
½ t Hot Sauce
Cumin to taste
Sea Salt to taste
Freshly Ground Black Pepper to taste

Mexican Shrimp Cocktail Sauce
Cold, Cooked Shrimp
Sugar-Free Picante Sauce or Fresh Salsa
Sugar Free Tomato Juice

Cilantro
Onion
Lemon or Lime Juice
Mix the salsa into the shrimp, until the shrimp are covered. Thin the sauce with the tomato juice and add the other ingredients to taste. Use cayenne or Tabasco and add a little Stevia if you don't like it tart.

Homemade BBQ Sauce
Liquid Smoke or 1 t Smoked Paprika or Chipotle Powder
1 Small Onion, Minced
1 Clove Garlic, Minced or ¼ t Garlic Powder
1 Small Can sugar-free (6 Oz) Tomato Paste
Stevia to taste
¼ C Sugar-Free Catsup (you can use the recipe in the Tips section for this)
3 T Mustard
1 T Worcestershire Sauce
Pinch of Ground Cloves
Hot Sauce to taste
1/2 C of Water
Pan-fry the onion in the Liquid Smoke over medium flame for about 4 minutes. Add garlic clove and stir. Add the remaining ingredients, including the water. Stir. Allow to simmer for 20-30 minutes. Stevia will tone down the spiciness if needed.

Homemade Salsa (great for steak salad or "taco salad" dressing)
½ small Tomato
2 slices Onion
Oregano
Chili Pepper
Red Pepper
Garlic Powder
Sea Salt
Freshly Ground Black Pepper
1 T Water
Add a dash of each spice to tomato and onion to taste and blend in food processor/blender with small amount of water. Don't forget that the tomato is your fruit serving.
5 minutes

Homemade Salsa, Too
Tomatoes
Cilantro
Cayenne
Lemon Juice
Apple Cider Vinegar
Sea Salt
Blend the tomatoes and add spices.

Green Salsa
Green Tomatoes
Salt
Garlic

Cilantro
Water
Blanch tomatoes and peel off skin. Boil until tender. Use food processor or blender to mix.

Beef Marinade
Bragg's Amino Acids
Any Spices you like

Homemade Taco Seasoning for Taco Salad
2 t Paprika
1 ½ t Sea Salt
1 t Onion Powder
1 t Chili Powder
1 ½ t Cumin
½ t Garlic Powder
For more kick, add a pinch of cayenne pepper. This is for one serving.

Blackened Chicken Seasoning
2 t Paprika
1 t Onion powder
1 t Garlic powder
1/4 t Cayenne (red) pepper
1/2 t White pepper
1/2 t Black pepper
1/2 t Sea Salt
1/2 t dried Thyme leaves
1/2 t dried Oregano leaves

Vegetables

Grilled Asparagus
Asparagus
Lemon Juice
Sea Salt
Fresh Cracked Black Pepper
Season asparagus with salt and pepper. Sprinkle with lemon juice and grill.
10 minutes

Asparagus Guacamole
12 spears Fresh Asparagus, trimmed and coarsely chopped
4 Green Onions, sliced, if mixing vegetables
¼ C Salsa (if mixing vegetables)
½ T Cilantro, chopped
2 cloves Garlic
Place the asparagus in a pot with enough water to cover. Bring to a boil, and cook 5 minutes, until tender but firm. Drain, and rinse with cold water. Place the asparagus, green onion and salsa if mixing vegetables, cilantro, garlic, and green onions in a food processor or blender, and process to desired consistency. Refrigerate 1 hour, or until chilled, before serving.
10 minutes, plus 1 hour refrigeration

Asparagus with Garlic and Lime

Medium Green Onion, minced, if mixing vegetables, or Onion Powder seasoning if not
1 bunch Fresh Asparagus spears, trimmed
¼ Lime, juiced
Sea Salt
Fresh Ground Black Pepper
Heat garlic and green onions or onion powder in a large skillet over medium heat for 1 to 2 minutes. Stir in asparagus spears; cook until tender, about 5 minutes. Squeeze lime over hot asparagus, and season with salt and pepper.
25 minutes

Marinated Asparagus

2 pounds fresh Asparagus, trimmed and cut into 2 1/2 inch pieces
1 ½ C Balsamic Vinaigrette dressing with no oil
2 t grated Lemon zest
¼ C chopped fresh Parsley
½ t Sea Salt
½ t Freshly Ground Black Pepper
Bring a large pot of salted water to a boil. Blanch asparagus just until tender, about 1 minute. Plunge into a bowl of cold water to cool. Drain asparagus and place in a large Ziploc plastic bag. Pour in vinaigrette and seal bag. Refrigerate at least 3 hours, turning bag occasionally.
Just before serving, drain asparagus, reserving vinaigrette. Arrange on a serving platter and sprinkle with lemon zest, parsley, salt, and pepper. Serve reserved vinaigrette in a small dish on the side.
35 minutes, plus 3 hours refrigeration

Roasted Roma Tomatoes with Garlic

8 Roma (plum) Tomatoes, halved
12 cloves Garlic, peeled
¼ C chopped Fresh Basil Leaves
Sea Salt
Freshly Ground Black Pepper
Preheat the oven to 400 degrees F (200 degrees C). Place the tomato halves in a shallow baking dish in which they can all fit in snugly side by side. Insert the whole cloves of garlic in between the tomatoes. Sprinkle with basil. Season with salt and pepper. Bake uncovered for 35 to 45 minutes, until tomatoes have softened and are sizzling in the pan with the edges slightly charred. Serve while hot.
1 hour

Baked Cherry Tomatoes with Garlic

1 pint Cherry Tomatoes
4 cloves Garlic, slivered
2 T Extra Virgin Olive Oil (Phase 3 only)
Kosher Salt (optional)
Preheat oven to 350 degrees F (175 degrees C). Cut a slit in one side of the cherry tomatoes, and insert a sliver of garlic into each. Arrange tomatoes in a single layer on a baking sheet. Drizzle with olive oil and sprinkle with salt. Bake tomatoes about 20 minutes in the preheated oven, until slightly shriveled. Serve warm.
30 minutes

Tomato Vinaigrette for Use on Meats

½ C chopped Tomatoes
2 T White Wine Vinegar
½ t dried or fresh Basil
½ t dried Thyme
½ t ground Mustard
In a blender or small food processor, blend or process the tomatoes, vinegar, basil, thyme, and mustard on medium to high speed, about 25 seconds or until well combined. To store, transfer to a jar with a tight-fitting cover and refrigerate for up to 2 days. Shake well before serving.
10 minutes

Melba Toast Bruschetta
Diced tomatoes
Onion
Cilantro
Balsamic Vinegar
Sea Salt to taste
Cut everything up, stir in balsamic vinegar and salt to taste. Top Melba toast with the mixture.
10 minutes

Baked/Grilled Onion
1 large Onion, peeled
Seasoned Salt to taste
Garlic Pepper to taste
Sea Salt
Freshly Ground Black Pepper
Set peeled onion upright on a sheet of foil. Make several deep slices in the onion without cutting completely through the onion. Sprinkle with seasoned salt, salt, pepper, and garlic pepper. Place the onion on a grill directly above a hot campfire or in the oven, and cook until the onion is soft, about 20 minutes.
25 minutes

Steamed Green Onions
12 Green Onions, rinsed, ends trimmed
2 cloves Garlic, minced
Sea Salt
Freshly Ground Black Pepper (optional)
Preheat a grill for medium-low heat. Cut a sheet of aluminum foil to about 12x15 inches. Arrange the green onions side by side in the center of the foil sheet. Sprinkle the onions evenly with the garlic, salt, and pepper. Keeping the green onions flat, fold the foil to make a sealed cooking pouch. Place the foil packet on the preheated grill away from the main heat source. Allow the green onions to steam 5 to 7 minutes.
10 minutes

Cabbage Rice/Noodle Alternative *A Tammy Recipe
½ head of cabbage finely chopped into rice sized or noodle size pieces
Spices
1 cup of water or chicken broth
　　Mexican style
1 cup tomatoes chopped
3 tablespoons tomato paste

2 tablespoons minced onion
1 clove of garlic crushed and minced
¼ teaspoon cayenne pepper or to taste
Pinch of oregano
Dash of Cumin to taste
Fresh chopped cilantro
Salt and pepper to taste

Italian style

1 cup tomatoes
3 tablespoons tomato paste
1/8 teaspoon fresh or dried oregano
1/8 teaspoon dried basil or 5 leaves fresh basil rolled and sliced
1 tablespoon minced onion
1 clove garlic crushed and minced
Pinch of marjoram
Salt and pepper to taste

Indian style

1/8 teaspoon curry
2 tablespoons minced onion
1 clove garlic crushed and minced
1/8 teaspoon cumin
Salt and pepper to taste

Oriental style

1/4 teaspoon ginger
3 tablespoons Bragg's liquid aminos
2 tablespoons lemon juice
3 tablespoons orange juice (optional)
2 tablespoons chopped onion
1 clove garlic crushed and minced

In a large frying pan sauté cabbage with a little water (vegetable or chicken broth may be substituted) and liquid ingredients. Add spices and cook until cabbage is tender adding water as necessary. For spaghetti style, serve Spaghetti-less meat sauce or marinara with Italian meatballs over steamed cabbage cut into noodle sized strips. Makes 1-2 servings (1 vegetable, 1 fruit if tomatoes are used)

Coleslaw

Grated Cabbage
Fresh Mint
Fresh Parsley
Red Wine Vinegar
Stevia
Onion Powder
Garlic Powder
Sea Salt
Freshly Ground Black Pepper

Combine the cabbage and herbs. Season with salt and pepper. Combine dressing ingredients in a small jar and shake. Combine with salad. Very refreshing.
10 minutes

Pickled Asparagus (this might be considered a cheat, however small, because it is pickled)
1 bunch fresh Asparagus

1 C Water
1 C Apple Cider Vinegar
4 cloves Garlic, crushed
1 Jalapeño Pepper, seeded and julienned
4 sprigs Fresh Thyme
2 T Old Bay seasoning
2 Bay leaves
1 t Sea Salt
6 whole Black Peppercorns

Trim the bottoms off of the asparagus, and pack loosely into a 1 quart jar. Combine the water, vinegar, garlic, Jalapeño, thyme sprigs, bay leaves, salt and whole peppercorns in a saucepan. Bring to a boil, and boil hard for 1 minute. Pour the hot liquid over the asparagus in the jar, filling to cover the tips of the asparagus. Cover, and cool to room temperature. Refrigerate 24 hours to meld.
15 minutes

Chilled Garlic Refrigerator Pickles *A Tammy Recipe
One medium cucumber sliced into rounds
4 cloves of garlic in thin slices
¼- ½ cup apple cider vinegar
3 tablespoons lemon juice
Salt

Mix liquid ingredients together. Salt cucumber slices well. Pack cucumber slices tightly into a small glass canning jar layering garlic slices in between layers. Pour apple cider vinegar and lemon juice into container until liquid covers the slices. Refrigerate overnight and enjoy. Pickles can be refrigerated for up to 4 days. Another variation of this is to marinate cucumber slices in salt, vinegar and garlic then put in a pickle press or using a weighted plate, press out excess liquid. Makes 1-2 servings (1 vegetable)

Seafood and Fish

Crab Cakes
3.5 ounces Crab Meat
4 ounces (or whatever you like) of Onion or Celery, your choice, chopped very finely
One portion of Melba toast ground into a "powder"
Sea Salt
Fresh Ground Black Pepper
Dash of Old Bay seasoning
Any other herbs to taste

Mix crab meat, vegetables, seasoning, and Melba toast powder. Fry with no oil or fat or water in the pan, until brown on one side. Flip and brown on other side.
20 minutes

Fillet of Cod with Fried Tomatoes
3.5 ounces Fillet of Cod
Tomatoes
Lemon Juice
Sea Salt
Fresh Ground Black Pepper

Sprinkle a bit of lemon juice on the cod and add a pinch of salt and pepper. Wrap fish in foil and let it cook in the oven for 30 minutes. In the meantime, fry the tomatoes on both sides in a special non-stick frying pan for a very short time without butter or oil, only with a little pinch of pepper and salt. Serve the tomatoes on a plate around the fillet of cod.
20 minutes

Whitefish with Onion and Tomatoes
Whitefish
1 Large Tomato, cut in chunks
Onion
Fat-Free Vegetable Broth
Lemon Juice
Garlic, minced
Sea Salt
Freshly Ground Black Pepper
Sauté onion in some vegetable broth and lemon juice. Add fish, garlic, tomatoes, salt, and pepper. Add tomatoes and cook for 2-3 minutes until cooked thoroughly. Phase 3 variation: Sauté onion in a little butter. Add fish, tomatoes, spices, and ½ C of half and half.
20 minutes

Grilled Mahi Mahi
Mahi Mahi
Fresh Lime Juice
Garlic, minced
Marinate fish in lime juice and garlic for about 5 minutes and then put it on the contact grill.
15 minutes

Shrimp Scampi
6 Jumbo Shrimp, frozen or thawed
¾ to 1 C Tomato
½ to 1 tsp Capers
½ tsp Onion Powder
½ tsp Garlic Powder
Juice from ½ Lemon
Fry the shrimp with the lemon juice. Add tomatoes and spices and cook until shrimp is opaque.
15 minutes

Shrimp and Tomato
Shrimp
Fresh Lemon Juice
Garlic, chopped
Red Pepper Flakes
½ Fresh Tomato
Cook the shrimp in a pan with a little water, lemon juice, garlic, pepper flakes, and tomato.
5 minutes

Shrimp/Fish and Asparagus
Shrimp or Fish
Asparagus
Garlic, minced

Fresh Lemon Juice
Spices of Choice
Grill shrimp or fish, with asparagus, garlic, lemon juice, and spices.
5 minutes

Cajun Shrimp
3.5 ounces Raw Shrimp
Onion
Garlic
Cayenne pepper
Freshly Ground Black Pepper
Paprika
Sea Salt
Lemon Juice
Sauté shrimp and spices with a little water until shrimp is opaque. Serve with salad or favorite vegetable.
15 minutes

Shrimp Ceviche
1-2 lbs. Shrimp, fresh or frozen, raw or cooked, peeled and deveined, tail-on or off
Juice of 2 large Lemons, freshly squeezed, about ¾ C to 1 C
Juice of 2-3 large Limes, freshly squeezed, about ¾ C to 1 C
1 T fresh Garlic, minced
1 Red Onion, finely chopped (about 1 C)
1-3 tablespoons Tabasco or pepper sauce (more or less to taste)
4 large Tomatoes, chopped (about 2-3 C) if mixing vegetables
2 Cucumbers, peeled and diced into 1/2 inch pieces (about 1 ½ C) if mixing vegetables
Fresh Cilantro, chopped (about ½ C)
Fresh Parsley, chopped (about ½ C)
Sea Salt to taste
Fresh Ground Black Pepper to taste
Thaw shrimp if frozen. If using raw shrimp, bring a pot of water to boil and cook the shrimp for a minute or two until it turns opaque white and reddish—do not over cook the shrimp as it will be too rubbery in texture. Rinse shrimp under cold water. Combine juices of lemons and limes in a large bowl (not metal) or large Ziploc baggie and add shrimp. Cover bowl or zip baggie and refrigerate for 30 minutes to marinade. Large shrimp could be cut into smaller chunks (remove tails if doing this) to speed up marinade time. Add to shrimp the Tabasco, garlic, onion, and pepper and mix. Return to refrigerator for another 30 minutes to let the flavors meld.
Before serving, add to the marinated shrimp mixture, cilantro, parsley, tomatoes (if mixing vegetables), and cucumbers (if mixing vegetables). If needed, add salt and pepper to taste.
1 hour

White Fish
3.5 ounces Any White Fish
Fresh Lemon Juice
Fresh Basil
Garlic, chopped
Oregano
Marinate fish in lemon juice, basil, garlic, and oregano for 10 minutes. Pan-fry or grill.

Grilled White Fish or Shrimp
3.5 ounces White Fish or Shrimp
Key Lime Juice
Garlic, minced
Sea Salt
Fresh Ground Black Pepper
Marinate fish in lime juice, lots of garlic, salt, and pepper for 20 minutes. Marinate shrimp 5 minutes. Grill it on a contact grill, but don't overcook. Shrimp can grill in 2 minutes.

Seabass with Garlic and Tomatoes
Garlic
Tomatoes, diced
Sea Salt
Fresh Ground Black Pepper
Brown both sides, then add the tomatoes and garlic.
20 minutes

Beef

Roast Beef and Cole Slaw Wrap
3.5 ounces Lean Sliced Roast Beef
Cabbage, Finely Shredded
Apple Cider Vinegar
Bragg's Amino Acids
Mustard Seed or Powder to taste
Garlic, minced
Celery Salt
Orange Flavored Stevia to taste
Sea Salt
Fresh Ground Black Pepper
Combine all except beef. Roll up the beef with the cole slaw inside and eat cold.

Roast Beef with Cucumber
3.5 ounces Grilled Roast Beef
1 Cucumber, grated coarsely
1 t Lemon Juice
Sea Salt
Freshly Ground Black Pepper
Roll up the slices of cooked roast beef and arrange them on a plate. Put the grated cucumber in a sieve and add a pinch of salt. Let the bitter liquid pour out of the cucumber for 10 minutes. Mix the cucumber with the lemon juice. Serve the cucumber together with the roast beef.

Burgers
3.5 ounces leanest Ground Beef
Garlic, chopped
Tomato (counts as your fruit)
Red Onion (optional)
Mix garlic with meat. Form into a patty and grill. Top with sliced tomato and red onion if mixing vegetables.

15 minutes

Burgers Too
1 lb leanest Ground Beef
1 t Freshly Ground Black Pepper
2 cloves Garlic, minced
1 or 2 T Onions, minced
¼ t Mustard Powder
Sprinkle of Oregano (optional)
Mix all ingredients in bowl. Measure out 3.5 ounce patties. Grill patties on medium heat until heated to 170-175. Turn only once to prevent dryness. Store leftover burgers in individual sealed bags in freezer until use.
30-45 minutes

Round Steak
Marinate top round steak in one of the marinades for up to 2 days and broil. Or slice it against the grain and stir fry it.

Slow Roasted Beef Brisket *A Tammy Recipe (A great crock pot recipe)
Lean beef brisket in weighed 100 gram increments (example 600 grams=6 servings)
2 cups chopped tomatoes (optional) (tomato used as a fruit)
4-6 stalks celery
3 tablespoons garlic powder
2 tablespoons onion powder
2 tablespoons paprika
1 onion chopped
5 cloves of garlic crushed and chopped
Cayenne pepper to taste
Chili pepper to taste
Salt and fresh ground black pepper to taste
Combine spices in a small bowl. Rub the mixture into the beef on all sides. Salt the meat liberally. Place the brisket in a crock pot. Fill about ½ ways with water. Add celery to the liquid and set crock pot on high for 30 minutes. Reduce heat to medium or low and allow to slow cook for 6-8 hours. Baste and turn the brisket periodically. You may add more of the spice mixture if you wish. Enjoy with horseradish sauce (page 44). Save the juices, skim the fat, and use to make flavorful sauces and dressings. Makes multiple servings (1 protein, 1 vegetable, 1 fruit) Phase 3 modifications: Sear on high heat in olive oil on each side before adding to crock pot. Horseradish sauce may be modified by adding mayonnaise or Greek yogurt instead of beef broth.

Beef/Chicken with Spinach/Onions and Garlic
3.5 ounces sliced lean Chicken or Steak
Fresh Spinach or Onions
Garlic
Sea Salt
Freshly Ground Black Pepper
Cook beef or chicken in a non-stick pan. Then, at the last minute, add in fresh spinach and seasoning. Or dice onions and throw them in a non-stick pan with your meat. Broth of some kind is helpful to season the meat as well. You could pour it in after the meat is cooked, to loosen the bits in the bottom of the pan and make an au jus to use for dipping the meat.

Chili

1 lb Veal, Buffalo, or Beef (very lean)
4 T Tomato Purée
9 large ripe Tomatoes, peeled and chopped
OR two 16 oz large cans of Glen Muir fire roasted Tomatoes
1 Onion, peeled and finely chopped
2 cloves of Garlic, crushed
1 t Chili Powder
Cayenne Pepper to taste
½ t Oregano
½ t Thyme
½ t Basil
Sea Salt to taste
Freshly Ground Black Pepper to taste
Brown meat with onions and garlic and drain meat of fat. Add 2 cans of 16 ounce Glen Muir fire roasted tomatoes and tomato paste. Simmer for an hour, spoon ¼ of the recipe into bowl, top with one crushed grissini bread stick or Melba toast.

Chili, Too

3.5 ounces leanest Ground Beef
7 ounces (or more) Tomatoes chopped
Chili Powder
Onion Powder
Garlic, chopped
Sea Salt
Freshly Ground Black Pepper
Cayenne
Simmer in covered saucepan.

Fajitas

Lean Sirloin or Chicken Breast
Yellow or White Onions
MSG-free Fajita seasoning
Sprinkle beef with fajita seasoning. Tenderize by beating or piercing. Sauté the onions and meat in a little water or chicken stock.
15 minutes

Chicken

Tangy Chicken

¼ C Apple Cider Vinegar
3 T Mustard Powder
3 cloves Garlic, peeled and minced
1 Lime, juiced
½ Lemon, juiced
½ C stevia
1 ½ t Sea Salt
Freshly Ground Black Pepper to taste
6 T Extra Virgin Olive Oil (Phase 3 variation)

6 Chicken Breasts or 12 Tenders
In a large glass bowl, mix the cider vinegar, mustard, garlic, lime juice, lemon juice, brown sugar, salt, and pepper. Whisk in the olive oil if on Phase 3. Place chicken in Ziploc bag with the mixture. Marinate 8 hours or overnight. Preheat an outdoor grill for high heat. Place chicken on the lightly oiled grill, and cook 6 to 8 minutes per side, until juices run clear. Discard marinade.

Hawaiian Chicken
3.5 oz Chicken, cut up into bite size pieces
Cabbage
½ clove Garlic, minced
Hawaiian seasoning
White Pepper to taste
Pan-fry until chicken is brown. Add ½ to 1/3 C water and let it deglaze. Add cabbage. The water in the pan quickly steams the cabbage to make it softer but still crunchy.
15 minutes

Sweet Lemon Chicken *A Tammy Recipe
100 grams thinly sliced chicken
½ lemon with rind
1 tablespoon Bragg's liquid aminos
½ cup chicken broth
1 cup water
Dash of cayenne pepper
Salt to taste
Stevia to taste (optional)
Slice up ½ lemons in to quarters and add to water. In a small saucepan boil lemon quarters until pulp comes out of the rind. Add broth, chicken, Bragg's, and spices and simmer on low heat until chicken is cooked and sauce is reduced by half. Deglaze periodically with water if necessary. Garnish with fresh lemon slices, lemon zest or mint. Serve over cabbage rice (recipe in vegetable section). Makes 1 serving (1 protein)

Shish Kabobs
Meat
Cherry Tomatoes
Onion
Asparagus
Herbs
Lemon Juice
Cube chunks of beef, fish, or chicken. Use cherry tomatoes, chunks of onion, and chopped asparagus. Put on skewer. Season with herbs and lemon juice and grill 15 minutes. Use just one of the vegetables with each meal.
20 minutes

Broiled Chicken
Chicken Breasts cut into 3.5 ounce servings
Apple Cider Vinegar
Lemon juice
Stevia
Spices

Marinate chicken in vinegar, lemon juice, and stevia. Add spices such as salt, pepper, curry, ginger, chili, and basil. Broil many of the servings together and bag them for later.
20 minutes

Grilled Chicken Breast
Fresh Rosemary
Fresh Garlic
Orange Zest
Coarse Salt
Pepper
Chop the rosemary, garlic and orange zest with the salt. Add the pepper. Rub mixture on raw chicken breast that has been seasoned with salt and pepper. Let it sit a while with the rub on it before cooking in a contact grill for 6 minutes
5 minutes

Broiled Chicken Breasts, Too
4 - 6 Chicken Breasts (no skin or fat)
Fat-Free Chicken Broth
Dried Parsley
Herbs De Provence or of your choice.
Turn burner on med-high. Add parsley and Herbs to the bottom of pan, coating evenly. Add chicken Breasts. Keep turning until seared. Things will start crystalizing on the bottom of pan, add about a ¼ C of chicken broth. Let boil until the liquid boils down. Repeat this process until chicken is done through and moist. I ususlly let it simmer adding more broth for at least an hour. Make as many as you can, so that you have chicken on hand. To reheat, put 3.5 ounces under the broiler for 5 minutes
1 hour

Melba Toast Bruschetta with Chicken
Chicken
Whole Wheat Melba Toast
Tomatoes
Basil
Oregano
Cilantro
Garlic
Freshly Ground Black Pepper (salt optional)
Juice of ½ Lemon
Chop desired quantity of tomatoes and mix with spices and lemon juice. Refrigerate mixture. Chop and sauté chicken and add spices to taste. Mix chicken in tomato mixture. Spoon on to Melba toast and eat the remainder with a spoon.
15 minutes

Chicken with Cucumbers
3.5 ounces Chicken (cooked)
1 Cucumber
Juice of 1 Lime
Peel the cucumber if you like and then slice thin. Slice the chicken into small pieces and add to cucumber.
5 min

Stir Fry
Chicken or Beef
Green Cabbage
Onion if mixing vegetables
Celery if mixing vegetables
Fat-Free Chicken Broth
Bragg's Amino Acids
Slice chicken and cabbage. Chop onion and celery small if mixing vegetables. Stir fry over med low with broth and liquid amino acids (tastes like soy sauce).
20 minutes

Chicken Chow Mein
Chopped Cabbage
3.5 ounces Chicken Breast
1- 2 T Onion
Pinch of Ginger
Sea Salt
Pinch of Stevia
Chop up cabbage, onions, and chicken. Place in a hot skillet and fry (keep it moving). Stir in spices. Cook until chicken is done, but not until the ingredients in the pan are dry.
10 minutes

Moo Shu Chicken
Chicken (julienne slice while frozen)
½ a small Green Cabbage sliced thin
½ C Fat-Free Chicken Broth
Bragg's Amino Acids
Cook cabbage with broth and amino acids on medium heat until wilted. Add chicken that has been sprayed with Bragg's into the pan and cook until chicken is done. Remove lid to evaporate all juice but don't burn.
10 minutes

Chicken Italiano
Chicken Breast
1 Tomato
Sea Salt
Garlic
Pepper
Italian seasoning
Chop up the tomato and the chicken breast into bite size chunks. Place in a hot frying pan and stir fry with all the seasonings.
15 minutes

Thanksgiving Chicken
Chicken Breast
Celery
Onion
Sage
Poultry seasoning
Sea Salt

Freshly Ground Black Pepper
Chop up chicken breast, celery and onion, stir fry in heated skillet, adding seasoning to taste.
15 minutes

Tomato Basil Chicken *A Tammy Recipe
100 grams cubed chicken
1 cup chopped tomato and juices
¼ cup water or chicken broth
2 tablespoons lemon juice
2 tablespoons chopped onion
1-2 cloves garlic sliced
5 leaves basil rolled and sliced
1/8 teaspoon oregano fresh or dried
¼ teaspoon garlic powder
1/8 teaspoon onion powder
Cayenne pepper to taste
Salt and pepper to taste
Lightly brown the chicken in small saucepan with lemon juice. Add garlic, onion, spices, and water. After chicken is cooked add fresh tomatoes and basil. Continue cooking for 5-10 minutes. Salt and pepper to taste, garnish with fresh basil. Makes 1 serving (1 protein, 1 fruit or vegetable)

Salads

Shrimp Salad
Marinate shrimp overnight in Old Bay seasoning and a splash of lime juice. Grill and serve over salad.

Taco Salad
7 ounces leanest Ground Beef
Mix spices (if possible) and set aside:
¾ t Cumin or to taste
¼ t Chili pepper or to taste
¼ t Red pepper or to taste
¼ t Oregano or to taste
¼ t Onion powder or to taste
¼ t Garlic or to taste
Sea Salt
Freshly Ground Black Pepper
¾ C Water
Lettuce
Brown meat, drain and pat with paper towel. Place meat back in pan. Sprinkle spices on top and add water. Heat to boiling and simmer for 15 minutes. Divide into 2 servings and serve over lettuce. I released 1 and 2 lbs on the days I made this.
20 minutes

Steak Salad
Steak
Lettuce OR Spinach OR Red Onion OR Radishes OR Red Cabbage
Tomato
Sea Salt

Freshly Ground Black Pepper
Grill steak until medium. Slice very thin. Chop vegetable of choice and serve room temp steak over salad. Season with pepper and salt.
20 minutes

Steak Salad, Too
Steak
Lettuce
Tomato
1 T Apple Cider Vinegar
Water
1 clove Garlic, minced
Sea Salt
Freshly Ground Black Pepper
Slice a grilled steak in very thin diagonal slices and serve over a bed of romaine with a tomato, using ACV, a little water, and garlic for dressing.
20 minutes

Spinach and Meat Salad
Baby Spinach
Chicken Breasts or Beef, grilled and chopped
Strawberries, sliced
¼ C Apple Cider Vinegar
2-3 packets Stevia
Sea Salt
Freshly Ground Black Pepper
Place clean spinach in a large salad bowl. Top with beef or chicken and strawberries. Mix vinegar with stevia and pour over salad.
5 minutes

Chicken and Salad
Chicken Breast, chopped small
Garlic
Oregano
Sea Salt
Freshly Ground Black Pepper
Cook in a non stick pan with garlic and oregano. Place over salad with a little Apple Cider Vinegar dressing.
20 minutes

Waldorf Salad
Lots of Celery, diced
1 Apple, diced
Chicken, cooked in cider vinegar and spices and diced
Juice of one or two Lemon wedges
1 or 2 T Apple Cider Vinegar
1 or 2 packets of Stevia
Cinnamon
Mix all together. Variation: Greens, Oranges, and Beef, with Orange flavored Stevia instead of the cinnamon.

5 minutes

Chicken and Tomatoes
Chicken Breasts
Grape tomatoes
Stevia
Basil
1 T Apple Cider Vinegar
1 clove Garlic, minced
Oregano
Lemon Juice to taste
Sea Salt
Freshly Ground Black Pepper
Cook chicken on contact grill and put the 3.5 ounce portions into individual Ziploc baggies and refrigerate. To prepare, dice a portion of chicken and put it in a bowl with a handful of grape tomatoes, cut in half. Mix it with stevia, basil, apple cider vinegar, garlic, oregano, and lemon juice.
25 minutes

Creole Chicken Salad
Chicken
Cajun Seasoning
Lettuce
Yellow Onion
Tomatoes
Sea Salt
Freshly Ground Black Pepper
Completely coat chicken breast with Cajun seasoning and grill. Slice and serve over salad, sprinkle with salt, pepper, and lemon juice if desired.
20 minutes

Chicken Salad (or Crab Salad, if you're eating crustaceans/ seafood)
3.5 ounces of Chicken or crab (real, not imitation, which has starch and sugar)
7 ounces Celery (or more)
Herbs
Sea Salt
Freshly Ground Black Pepper
Dice chicken or crab very fine. Chop celery. Add dash of mustard, salt, pepper, cayenne, vinegar, and whatever herbs you like (savory and parsley work well). Mix all the ingredients together in a bowl. Serve chilled.
5 minutes

Chicken Strawberry Spinach Salad
3.5 ounces Chicken Breast, cut into bite-size pieces
½ t Garlic Powder
½ Lime, juiced
½ t ground Ginger
2 C fresh Spinach, stems removed
4-6 fresh Strawberries, sliced
1 Grissini, crumbled
Sea Salt

80

Freshly Ground Black Pepper to taste
Heat chicken in skillet, season with garlic powder and cook 10 minutes on medium on each side or until juices run clear. Set aside. In a bowl, mix lime juice and ginger. Arrange spinach on serving dishes. Top with chicken and strawberries, sprinkle with crumbled breadstick and drizzle with dressing. Season with pepper to serve.
25 minutes

Tomato Salad
Cherry Tomatoes
Fresh Basil
Red Wine Vinegar
Stevia
Sea Salt
Freshly Ground Black Pepper
Cut tomatoes in half. Add chopped basil. Season with Salt and Pepper, Make a bit of "dressing" with red wine vinegar and stevia. You could add garlic powder or crushed fresh garlic if you want to. Let stand at room temperature for a few minutes before serving to blend flavors
5 minutes

Tomato Salad, Too
Chopped Tomato
Green Onion
Cilantro
Jalapeño
Sea Salt
Freshly Ground Black Pepper
You can add lemon if you want to. You have to taste it and occasionally add more tomato to cut the spiciness, or add more jalapeño.
5 minutes

Soups

Asparagus Soup
Asparagus, broken into pieces
Lemon Juice
ACV
Garlic Powder
2 C Fat-Free Chicken Broth
Sea Salt and freshly ground Black Pepper to taste
Lightly steam with lemon juice, apple cider vinegar, and garlic powder sprinkled on chicken broth. Add extra water to have enough broth. Blend in blender on high; heat, add salt and pepper to taste.
Variation: Add the T of milk that's allowed daily and make a "cream of asparagus" soup.

Tomato Basil Soup
3 large ripe Tomatoes, peeled and chopped, or one 16 oz large can of fire roasted tomatoes
1 Onion, peeled and finely chopped
1 clove Garlic, crushed
Fresh Basil leaves
1 can Fat-Free Chicken or Vegetable Stock

1 T Tomato Purée
Sea Salt and freshly ground Black Pepper to taste
Stir in 1 serving (3.5 oz.) chicken to make it a main dish. If prepared with vegetable stock, it will be suitable for vegetarians.

French Onion Soup
2 cans Fat-Free Chicken Stock
1 Beef Bouillon Cube
1 dash Worcestershire Sauce
2 medium Onions, sliced thin
2 packets Stevia
Sea Salt
Freshly Ground Black Pepper to taste
Stir-fry the onions with a little of the chicken stock, salt, and pepper until soft/browned.
Bring the rest of the ingredients to a boil in separate pot, then add the onions and let simmer for about 20 minutes.
30 minutes

Shrimp Gumbo (One of my favorites)
3.5 ounces Shrimp
7 ounces (or more) chopped Celery
Dash of Cayenne Pepper
Sea Salt
Freshly Ground Black Pepper
 (if you treat tomato as a fruit, use 1 ounce of chopped tomato) Note: you can also make this with full serving of tomato instead of with the celery. Just add celery seed to get the celery flavor. Put everything in saucepan with a dash of Apple Cider Vinegar and cover until the celery is slightly cooked and shrimp are opaque.

Spicy Chicken Soup
2 - 3 lbs Chicken Breast cut into squares
Worcestershire sauce - sugar free, fat free
Tabasco sauce
Homemade Fat-Free Chicken Stock
2 Tomatoes, blended first with 1/2 ltr water
½ clove Garlic
Lemon or Lime juice
Any of the following: Parsley, Dill, Cilantro, Sea Salt and Pepper to taste.
2 ½ liters Water
Boil for about 20 minutes.

Chicken Celery Soup
Chicken Breast
Celery
Onion Powder
Italian seasoning
Pinch cayenne
Salt and Pepper
Garlic if desired
Use water to cover. Simmer all together. Use at least one stalk of celery for each 3.5 ounces of meat

15 minutes

Desserts

Strawberry Smoothie
Strawberries
Ice
Stevia
Add some fresh squeezed lemon juice and a little water for a delicious 'daiquiri'. Put it in a goblet to make yourself feel special.

Apple Pie
Apple
¼ tsp Cinnamon
Dash Stevia
Cut apple into slices (pie style). Remove the core and seeds but don't peel. Arrange in a serving size Pyrex or ceramic bowl. Sprinkle with cinnamon and stevia. Bake in 375 degree oven for 20 minutes. Use the liquid English Toffee flavored stevia or Pumpkin Pie spice for variety. Or coat it with lemon and sprinkle with allspice.

Strawberry Pops or Sorbet
Fresh Strawberries
Lemon Juice
Stevia
Fresh Mint (optional)
Puree ingredients and pour into pop molds or C. Freeze until firm.
5 minutes

Miscellaneous

Spanish Omelette
3 Egg Whites
1 Whole Egg
Cumin
Onion, diced
Tomato, diced
Sea Salt to taste
Freshly Ground Black Pepper to taste
Use different herbs and/or veggie to change this up. Tomato counts as fruit.

HCG Recipe Substitutions
Bacon = Liquid Smoke

Step 26 – Plan your Phase 2 meals
Plan your Phase 2 meals for the first week using the Meal Planning Auto Calorie Calculator Spreadsheet found in the files section of the group.

Sample Menus

Phase 2 Sample Menu 1

Breakfast: ½ grapefruit
Coffee with vanilla stevia and 1 T milk
Lunch: 3.5 oz grilled chicken with lettuce salad using herbs, salt, and apple cider vinegar
Afternoon snack: 6 strawberries
Dinner: 6 grilled shrimp with garlic salt and Cajun spices with steamed spinach with lemon juice

Phase 2 Sample Menu 2

Breakfast: Orange	62 calories
Snack: Raw Cabbage with vinegar in a slaw	35 calories
Lunch: 3.5 ounces Chicken sautéed with Cabbage	155 calories
Snack: Tomato sliced with salt and pepper	36 calories
Dinner: 3.5 ounces Chicken sautéed with Tomato and Cajun seasoning	141 calories
Snack: Apple	67 calories
Total:	496 calories

Phase 2 Sample Menu 3

Lunch: Pink Lady Apple, Roasted Tomatoes, 3.5 oz White Fish
Dinner: Honeycrisp Apple, Romaine Lettuce, 3.5 oz Ground Sirloin

Phase 2 Sample Menu 4

Breakfast: Coffee with 1 T milk and Cinnamon Liquid Stevia
Snack: ½ grapefruit
Lunch: Shrimp with salad and Melba toast
Dinner: Chicken and asparagus with grissini breadstick
Snack: Baked Apple with Cinnamon Liquid Stevia

How many ounces is 100 grams for the protein serving?

100 grams equals 3.5273962 ounces.

Are foods weighed raw or cooked to measure the portions?

You weigh it raw, but not frozen, so you count the calories based on that. Yes, you are eating it cooked, but the cooked weight would be different and you would have to use calories per cooked ounce rather than calories per raw ounce. Cooking doesn't alter the calories. What I mean is, if you get 104 calories for your 100 g of meat raw, after you cook it, it will have the same amount of calories as it did raw. It will weigh less, but have the same number of calories, which explains why cooked meat has more calories per gram or ounce than raw does. For example, 100 grams of RAW chicken weighs 86 grams after cooking and 106 grams when frozen, so different caloric counts are given per ounce for different states.

Why can't we eat turkey on Phase 2?

The short answer is: Because you will not lose weight with it. It will stall your reducing and you might even gain. All of us have found that out from experience, but if you don't believe Dr S's 40 years of experience when he wrote the manuscript, have at it. You will find out the same that we did. Dr S is right. He didn't explain the reasons for every single rule he had, but those rules came from actual experience with patients on the diet.

What are considered white fish that ARE allowed in Phase 2?

Ayr, Catfish, Cod, Coley, Flounder, Flying fish, Haddock, Hake, Halibut, Hoki, John dory, Kalabasu, Ling, Monk fish, Parrot fish, Plaice, Pollack, Pomfret, Red & grey mullet, Red fish, Red Snapper, Rohu, Rock Salmon/Dogfish, Sea bass, Sea bream, Shark, Skate, Sole, Tilapia, Turbot, and Whiting Cod

What are considered fatty fish NOT allowed in Phase 2?

Anchovies, Bloater, Cacha, Carp, Eel, Herring, Hilsa, Jack fish, Katla, Kipper, Mackerel, Orange roughy, Pangas, Pilchards, Salmon, Sardines, Sprats, Swordfish, Trout, Tuna, and Whitebate

Can I eat shellfish in Phase 2 or will it stall my weight reduction?

Lobster, crab, and shrimp are clearly allowed by Simeons in the original manuscript and I have eaten them without incident. KT left them out for other reasons, not weight reduction reasons.

Should I eat the grissini or Melba toast that Dr. Simeons allows, but Trudeau does not?

It's a personal choice. Some have problems with starch and don't want to deal with eating a small quantity of it because it triggers their cravings. Someone else said they didn't feel satisfied until they added the grissini/Melba toast. Twenty calories of Wasa can be substituted for these as well. Some don't eat it because they would rather eat other things using those calories. Some are gluten-intolerant. Gluten-free grissini can be found on-line or at Kroger under the Glutino brand. However, there are some things to consider here. Dr S said on page 63 that "When local conditions or the feeding habits of the population make changes necessary it must be borne in mind that the total daily intake must not exceed 500 Calories if the best possible results are to be obtained, that the daily ration should contain 200 grams of fat-free protein and a very small amount of starch." Some have reported that they became unable to eat normal amounts of starch in P4 after leaving it out of P2 while on hCG.

How many ounces of vegetables can I have per day?

There really is no limit on the veggies, even though KT stated to eat a "handful" at each meal. The only limit is the total of 500 calories/day. So you can have a huge amount of veggies (since they are so low in calories) to make up the difference, up to a total of 500 calories for the day. Use the calories found in your two proteins, your two fruits, your two Melba/grissini/Wasas (if chosen) and then subtract that from 500 and make up the rest in vegetables.

"Pounds and Inches" states NOT to mix vegetables, but "Weight Loss Cure" states DO?

The Weight Loss Cure book has a typographical error. A couple of pages later he says you can't. He put the word DO in capital letters and it appears he meant to add the word NOT to it. That said, some people have reported mixing vegetables without a weight reduction stall occurring.

Can I eat cherry tomatoes and grape tomatoes instead of regular tomatoes?

Those varieties are sweeter and have different nutrient counts than heirloom or Roma tomatoes. An ounce of tomato has 1.1 grams of carbs, .7 grams of sugar and 5 calories. But, an ounce of grape tomatoes has 2 grams of carbs, 1 gram of sugar and 8 calories; and an ounce of cherry tomatoes has 1.7 grams of carbs, 1 gram of sugar, and 8 calories. You may stall on these types.

Do I have to eat different foods at each meal?

This is a common misconception. Dr Simeons didn't say that. Here is what he said on page 62: "American beef has almost double the caloric value of South Italian beef, which is not marbled with fat. This marbling is impossible to remove. In America, therefore, low-grade veal should be used for one meal and fish (excluding all those species such as herring, mackerel, tuna, salmon, eel, etc., which have a high fat content, and all dried, smoked or pickled fish), chicken breast, lobster, crawfish, prawns, shrimps, crabmeat or kidneys for the other meal."

He didn't say that you had to have something different for each meal. He said that if you use what was typical American beef in 1971 for one meal, you should use a lower fat protein source for the other meal and not beef again.

Can I try eating "x" while on Phase 2? It has the same calories as "y."

If you haven't already, read the Simeons protocol, in which he addresses trying to substitute one food for another based on calories. Page 62 states: "The most tiresome patients are those who start counting Calories and then come up with all manner of ingenious variations which they compile from their little books. When one has spent years of weary research trying to make a diet as attractive as possible without jeopardizing the loss of weight, culinary geniuses who are out to improve their unhappy lot are hard to take." I agree with him.

Dr. S goes on to say that, "Every item in the list is gone over carefully, continually stressing the point that no variations other than those listed may be introduced. All things not listed are forbidden, and the patient is assured that nothing permissible has been left out."

I hope this explains why I will not answer questions about deviating from the diet given in Dr. Simeons' protocol. Please don't email to ask that kind of question. The protocol works. It will be true to you if you are true to it.

Please don't ask questions that have already been answered in this book, such as "Can I eat this or that?" or "Can I use this product or that?" and especially not "Can I use this medication or that?" I am a dieter, not a doctor, and pretty much of a purist where this protocol is concerned.

Tips

Crush Melba toast or grissini on top of dishes for a crouton effect.

Raw, unfiltered, unpasteurized, Apple Cider Vinegar with the "mother" does not feed Candida.

Use a piece of foil to line the contact grill (George Foreman type). Food doesn't stick to the grill and there's no cleanup.

For those having trouble drinking water, try a few drops of flavored stevia in water to add some flavor and variety.

When covering and cooking after adding veggies, be sure to turn the heat very low to prevent a boiled texture.

Instead of ketchup, try this recipe. Boil tomatoes for 10 minutes. Put in food processor with garlic, spices, and a little sea salt. Keep in the refrigerator. Add Stevia if you want a sweeter flavor.

Try 2 teaspoons Apple Cider Vinegar in a very large glass of very cold water with some Stevia as an "ACV cocktail". Almost like lemonade - sweet and sour mixed together with a hint of apple in the background. I actually enjoy starting my day with the cocktail as well as at least one other time during the day. Try it; you might like it!

Thaw frozen shrimp quickly by soaking it in cold water.

Split your meals up. Just because you are allowed 3.5 oz of protein doesn't mean you have to eat it all at "Lunch" or "Dinner". Same with the veggies, fruit, and Grissini or Melba toast. Space it out so that you can eat every couple hours, but keep in mind not to exceed the allowances of 7 oz. of protein and 500 calories total per day. And if you have any blood sugar stabilization issues, it could help to eat a little of your protein with the fruit or grissini rather than having them alone.

If you're a coffee drinker, sip your cup throughout the day. I don't need mine much in the morning, but after 4 pm (the postprandial dip), I use the coffee (and Yerba Mate Royale) to quell hunger pangs.

Leanest Beef Cuts	Leanest Veal Cuts
top round (inside round steak)	leg cutlet
eye of round	blade steak
round tip or bottom round	rib roast
shank or arm	shoulder steak
sirloin steak	loin chop
rump roast	
top loin	
t-bone	
tenderloin or filet	

Bison (buffalo) is leaner than beef, and many have used it without problems.

For dessert, have strawberries with a little dark chocolate stevia.

Keep an apple or slices in the car for a breakfast or snack.

It's actually very easy to hold a job while doing this protocol. Always take a cooler in the car with chopped veggies, fruits, and proteins. Also lots of water, packets of teas, etc.

Precook all your meals. I cook up my chicken, steak, and fish, weigh them, and freeze some and refrigerate others so I'm ready to go. After purchasing my fresh meat regardless of what it is, I weigh it raw and put it in a sandwich size zipper baggie and I am portioned out. Then I put all the same cuts into a gallon size baggie in the freezer. So I end up with a few gallon size baggies labeled Chicken, Tenderloin, Eye of Round, etc. Just make sure your gallon size bags are the strong freezer type.

On Phase 3, use parmesan cheese (the kind you sprinkle over your spaghetti) to thicken sauces or gravies instead of the flour or cornstarch that we cannot have during the stabilization period. It works really well and tastes good, too.

Cilantro makes almost anything taste either Mexican or Thai!

And finally, a suggestion if you must cheat. Slice a cucumber very thin and soak in some apple cider vinegar and salt. Store in a tightly sealed jar in the refrigerator. You can also do this with fresh squeezed lemon juice instead of the ACV. You can use these as your veggie for a meal or even to accent a bland meal with a tiny cheat by taking one very thin (1/8 inch or less) slice of cucumber and squeezing out the vinegar or lemon juice if it is too tart for you, then dicing it extra fine into tiny little bits. Just that little bite of cucumber tastes like a pickle and gives a little sizzle to a meal. This little cheat has helped me stay away from giving in to bigger ones.

Step 27 – Set interim goals for yourself for motivation.

Set interim goals for yourself so that you can celebrate your success along the way.

Help! I need motivation to keep from cheating.

Here are some of the ways that I keep myself motivated to keep myself from cheating on this plan:

1. Setting the interim goals gives me a sense of satisfaction when I reach them. If I'm tempted by some food that someone else is eating, I think about how much I want to reach the next goal.
2. When I am tempted, I write down that food in my diet journal in a place specifically for my next load day foods. Then I know that I can have it and I will have it again, just not right now.
3. I'm really not that hungry on hCG (and this coming from someone who used to eat 3000 - 5000 calories a day).
4. I see results almost every morning on the scale.
5. It's relatively short term in any one of my rounds – I know that before long I'll be able to have a lot more food than I am having on the VLCD and different foods than allowed on VLCD.
6. I make a list of the things that I look forward to the most that I will enjoy when I am at goal...but NOT FOODS, all the wonderful experiences and feelings that I can have at a lower weight.

Another link to help with daily motivation: **http://tinyurl.com/motivator1**

Another motivator is using a ticker in your email signature to remind you of how far you have come. **http://tinyurl.com/motivator2** has free tickers that you can use. Here are some instructions: When using Yahoo email, I set my email setting to Rich Text (to the right of the Subject Line). Then I go to Options (above the email tab, between Mobile and Help) then Mail Options. Next, I select Signature, then select Rich Text for the Signature, then I copy in the HTML code under my signature and Save Changes. Every few days, I update the ticker by clicking on my ticker in a previous email to go to the website, enter my password, and update my weight, which automatically updates any previous signature as well.

Step 28 – If doing this on your own, on the first day of Phase 2, mix the hCG and store it properly.

Mixing hCG

I just got my hCG. It looks like it is liquid. Why does everything mention powder?

hCG is shipped as powder, but in glass ampoules or vials along with more ampoules or vials of liquid solvent, which are the same size as the powdered hCG. You may be looking at the solvent, or not looking closely enough at the powder to realize that it isn't liquid in the glass ampoule/vial.

I just got my hCG. It states on the label "For Injections Only". I want to use it for sublingual dosing. Can I?

All hCG states that. That is what all of the members of my support group use for sublingual mixing and dosing with no issues reported. I don't think that the molecule from any SL mix would be absorbed completely whole, just as Dr B theorized, nor do I believe that it stays in the body as long, so dosage is increased and two doses per day are used to compensate for these sublingual dosing characteristics.

Helpful Notes Regarding the Preparation of hCG Diet Shots

1 ml = 1 cc, which are both measures of volume, NOT a particular dosage of hCG
IU = international units, which are measures of dosage of hCG
Don't forget to keep hCG refrigerated after mixing. It can only stay potent for two or three days at room temperature.

Preparing hCG injections for weight reduction

If your physician or clinic has given you a prescription for hCG for your weight reduction protocol, this section may help with mixing and storing the hCG and self-administration of hCG shots.

On page 128 of Weight Loss Cure, KT states that hCG needs to be mixed fresh every day. Is that true?

It is impossible to mix daily unless you are sharing what you mix among many people. The hCG doesn't come in small enough doses. The hCG probably stays potent at least 30 days after mixing, as long as it is kept refrigerated. KT is the only one to state that you must mix daily. Dr B mixes sublingual twice a week for his patients, according to one of the people on my support group that sees him.

Can I re-use syringes or needles?

They're cheap, so I would never scrimp when it comes to my health and sterility of injections. Depending on where you live, you may be able to buy them at a pharmacy. There are many other reasons that people self-inject besides being a diabetic. I have a friend who gives herself B-12 injections every week and buys her needle/syringe combos at a pharmacy. At Costco, a box of 100 costs $27.50. Most people buy enough to last and buy extra needles to change to after drawing up the hCG, so that they are not injecting with a needle dulled by piercing the rubber top of the vial.

How do I decide on a dosage?

Discuss the dosage amount for your protocol with your health provider. Dr. Simeons' original hCG diet protocol calls for 125 IU daily doses. Kevin Trudeau has published a different protocol, calling for 175 IU to 200 IU dependent on various factors, including the amount of weight that needs to be released.

Remember that Dr S instructs to skip an injection 1 day per week on the 43-day protocol in order to lessen the potential for immunity, and the skipped day should always remain on the same day of the week. He also states that each dose should be given as near to the same time each day as possible.

The hCG freeze-dried powder is measured in IU. It can be diluted to any concentration desired, depending upon how much solvent is added. All of the dilution measurements are in either cc or ml, which are one and the same. e.g. If 1500 IU hCG is diluted with a total of 12 cc (ml) of appropriate solvent (bacteriostatic water for injection or bacteriostatic sodium chloride for injection), it will yield a concentration of: 1500 IU / 12 cc = 125 IU per cc. In reverse, if someone has a 1500 IU vial and wants to mix a certain dosage (based upon injecting 1 cc/day), let's say 150 IU per day, then 1500 IU is divided by 150 IU/day to equal 10 days. That would mean a total of 10 cc (ml) of solvent is added to the hCG freeze-dried powder (usually a person would dissolve the powder using 1 cc of solvent and then add the rest of the solvent to the sterile vial after that).

Dosage can be adjusted up or down, depending on how a body reacts to the dosage. Most people in my support group use logic and pick a starting point. If someone is releasing weight and not hungry, then that level is working. If someone is not releasing weight (absent other factors such as cheating, sneaky sugar, accidental exposure to fats, etc.), or is hungry past the first week, then that person might need to up the dose, or if already high, possibly lower it for better results. When changing doses, most people wait 3 days before switching again because it takes 3 days to kick in.

Just realize that if a large amount of hCG is mixed all at once, some of that large batch might have to be thrown away at some point as the hCG becomes less and less effective as it deteriorates over a period of time – a good reason for people to mix their own in as small a batch as possible, so that it will be as fresh as possible.

Mixing for Injections

First, I would make sure there are enough ampoules or vials of freeze-dried powdered hCG on hand to complete the number of days that you plan to do, although you won't be mixing it all at once. Running out of hCG in the middle of a 43-day round would be an awful surprise when you are on a roll with the weight reduction going well! There should be an expiration date printed on the container of freeze-dried powdered hCG. I always check this date first and replace it if expired. Before reconstituting hCG, I store the solvent in the refrigerator to ensure that the hCG is cooled as soon as the solvent hits it and it becomes liquid, to preserve the potency.

Most people gather all of their supplies before beginning. Required mixing materials: hCG in freeze-dried powder concentrate, injection safe appropriate solvent, syringes for mixing with replacement needles, alcohol pads, and an empty sterile glass vial. The hCG is normally provided with a 1 ml ampoule of appropriate liquid solvent to be mixed with it; however, this amount is not sufficient for the hCG weight reduction shots. If getting a 10,000 IU vial of Novarel from the local pharmacy, a 30 ml vial of bacteriostatic water is included with it. Purchasing a larger vial of injection safe appropriate solvent is required for most other brands. Appropriate solvent that is safe for injecting can be found at your pharmacy if you have a prescription or at the same web sites that sell supplies. A glass vial is recommended for your hCG. For 175 IU doses, 30 ml of water is needed. Appropriate solvent preserves the mixed hCG for up to one month, IF KEPT REFRIGERATED. If there is solution remaining after your entire cycle of weight reduction is complete, it should be discarded. Its potency will become depleted over time and the bio-active potency life of hCG after it has been reconstituted and suspended in solution is uncertain.

Another factor that relates to potency, effectiveness, and bio-active life is that hCG should be handled gently at all times. In other words, no shaking of the mix, no squirting diluent quickly into the hCG or solution, and you don't want to see bubbles or foaming. If you do, you probably have damaged the hCG, meaning that it might not work at all, because the molecule has been damaged and is no longer whole and intact. hCG is a very large and fragile molecule and the bonds can be broken more easily than some other proteins.

90

Mixing Preparation

hCG weight reduction shots are prepared in a sterile environment. The area should be cleaned with bleach or alcohol and left to *air dry*. Mixing materials should be laid out in the sterile environment and hands should be washed with anti-bacterial soap. Hands should be dried with paper towels.

Opening the glass ampoule of the hCG powder concentrate

The top of the ampoule must be cleaned with an alcohol pad. When breaking an ampoule, great force or tight squeezing are not needed to break it cleanly in the smallest part of the neck. If you look at the ampoule, you should see a small black dot at the neck (the bumped-in spot between the upper portion and the lower bottle portion). Before I switched to an ampoule opener, I put mine in a washcloth (to protect my hands) and just positioned it so the black dot is in the front under my thumb and held the lower portion in one hand and the upper portion in the other hand and break the ampoule at that point by applying pressure on the upper portion in a backwards direction (away from the black dot). If you look closely, you'll see a little chip, score, or cut in the glass there. They give you a start by making a weak point in the ampoule without violating its sterility, so that someone can just apply pressure so that it "snaps" at that point like a twig. The black dot is there to show where the "chip" or break point is. The ampoule can be gently snapped in half as if it were a twig, while taking great care not to allow any bits of glass to fall into the ampoule. This is easiest to do while keeping a thumb toward the **bottom end** of the ampoule. If I tried to put pressure too close to the "neck" of the bottle, it wouldn't break open. Once you get the first one open, you will get the hang of it. It really does just "snap" like a little twig. You could practice on the liquid ampoules that came with it. Also, the opened ampoule has sharp edges. When handling the ampoule after opening it, I used a small plastic bag for disposal. Ampoule openers are available: **http://tinyurl.com/ampopener http://tinyurl.com/ampopener2**

Some recommend using a filter syringe during the mixing process in case any microscopic bits of glass get into the mixture. In my experience, it is not difficult to avoid having bits of glass fall into the solution. If you are concerned, filter syringes are available: **http://tinyurl.com/syringefilter**

A large 30 cc syringe is used for the mixing process. Also, using a larger gauge needle just for mixing makes it much easier to withdraw several ccs of appropriate solvent and reduces the chances of foaming. The needles of the other smaller syringes will be too short to get near the bottom of the ampoule/vial when withdrawing the solution. Don't worry; you will not be using these larger syringe(s) for your injections. Following are directions that many of my support group members have used:

- o   Flip the outer metal top off of the appropriate solvent.
- o   Sterilize the rubber top of the 30 cc sterile appropriate solvent vial with a new alcohol pad.
- o   Sterilize the rubber top of a new sterile glass vial with a new alcohol pad.
- o   Using a 30 cc syringe, draw the indicated amount of sterile appropriate solvent into the syringe.
- o   Replace the needle.
- o   Inject only 1 cc of this sterile appropriate solvent into the hCG ampoule, SLOWLY down the side of the glass, not allowing the needle to touch the glass. You don't want bubbles. If the needle touches the glass, replace the needle before continuing to the next step. The powder will dissolve almost immediately, with a gentle swirling of the vial. DO NOT SHAKE. Handle the hCG carefully.
- o   With a new 3 cc syringe, draw the 1 cc of hCG out of the ampoule.

Here are some tips for doing this step:
When I went to withdraw the hCG, I quickly realized that the needle was too short to reach the bottom of the ampoule. The ampoules are 2" deep and I had 1" needles. So I had to tilt the ampoule on its side to get the mixture close enough to withdraw and it took some time to get it all in the syringe. You

don't want to miss any because it will affect the dosage formula of the mixture. I discussed the issue with an RN and she confirmed that you CAN invert the ampoule (turn it upside down) WITH the hCG in it and the mix will not come out. It is simple physics. The design of the ampoule creates a vacuum in the ampoule that prevents the mix from draining out. It sounds crazy and it is scary to do because you don't want to lose the hCG. But it works. NEVER insert AIR into the ampoule like you do when you withdraw from a vial. The inserted air breaks the vacuum and all the liquid will come out very fast. Just put the point of the needle in far enough to be in the liquid. Then draw back VERY SLOWLY. At the end, you may need to tilt the ampoule to get the very last drops. Again, practice with the solvent ampoule FIRST until you are comfortable with the process.

o   Withdraw every drop of the hCG solution and inject it into the empty glass vial.
o   Inject the rest of the sterile appropriate solvent from the large 30 cc syringe into the new sterile glass vial containing the 1cc of hCG that you just finished mixing.
o   Each day you will take a 1 cc injection from this vial until it is time to mix again or until you reach the last day of your round of injections.

It seems that lots of folks are challenged when it comes to figuring out the amount of liquid to use in a mix. It's just basic math, though. For example, 5000 divided by 125 = 40. So if you add 40 ml solvent to the hCG, and do 1 ml per day, that would be a 125 IU dose. If you want to cut that amount (not the dose) in half and only take .5 ml each day, then you would halve the amount of liquid you put in. However, because so many seem to need help, I created the table below to help you.

Pounds and Inches Mixing Calculator

Ampoule Size (IU)	Desired Dosage Volume (ml)	Desired Dosage Strength (IU)	Amount of Liquid to Add (ml)	Number of Doses That Will Result
10000	1.0	125	80.0	80.0
10000	1.0	133	75.2	75.2
10000	1.0	150	66.7	66.7
10000	1.0	166	60.2	60.2
10000	1.0	175	57.1	57.1
10000	1.0	200	50.0	50.0
10000	1.0	225	44.4	44.4
10000	1.0	250	40.0	40.0
10000	0.5	125	40.0	80.0
10000	0.5	133	37.6	75.2
10000	0.5	150	33.3	66.7
10000	0.5	166	30.1	60.2
10000	0.5	175	28.6	57.1
10000	0.5	200	25.0	50.0
10000	0.5	225	22.2	44.4
10000	0.5	250	20.0	40.0
5000	1.0	125	40.0	40.0
5000	1.0	133	37.6	37.6
5000	1.0	150	33.3	33.3
5000	1.0	166	30.1	30.1
5000	1.0	175	28.6	28.6
5000	1.0	200	25.0	25.0
5000	1.0	225	22.2	22.2

Ampoule Size (IU)	Desired Dosage Volume (ml)	Desired Dosage Strength (IU)	Amount of Liquid to Add (ml)	Number of Doses That Will Result
5000	1.0	250	20.0	20.0
5000	0.5	125	20.0	40.0
5000	0.5	133	18.8	37.6
5000	0.5	150	16.7	33.3
5000	0.5	166	15.1	30.1
5000	0.5	175	14.3	28.6
5000	0.5	200	12.5	25.0
5000	0.5	225	11.1	22.2
5000	0.5	250	10.0	20.0
2000	1.0	125	16.0	16.0
2000	1.0	133	15.0	15.0
2000	1.0	150	13.3	13.3
2000	1.0	166	12.0	12.0
2000	1.0	175	11.4	11.4
2000	1.0	200	10.0	10.0
2000	1.0	225	8.9	8.9
2000	1.0	250	8.0	8.0
2000	0.5	125	8.0	16.0
2000	0.5	133	7.5	15.0
2000	0.5	150	6.7	13.3
2000	0.5	166	6.0	12.0
2000	0.5	175	5.7	11.4
2000	0.5	200	5.0	10.0
2000	0.5	225	4.4	8.9
2000	0.5	250	4.0	8.0
1500	1.0	125	12.0	12.0
1500	1.0	133	11.3	11.3
1500	1.0	150	10.0	10.0
1500	1.0	166	9.0	9.0
1500	1.0	175	8.6	8.6
1500	1.0	200	7.5	7.5
1500	1.0	225	6.7	6.7
1500	1.0	250	6.0	6.0
1500	0.5	125	6.0	12.0
1500	0.5	133	5.6	11.3
1500	0.5	150	5.0	10.0
1500	0.5	166	4.5	9.0
1500	0.5	175	4.3	8.6
1500	0.5	200	3.8	7.5
1500	0.5	225	3.3	6.7
1500	0.5	250	3.0	6.0

Mixing for Sublingual

Many recipes for sublingual hCG that are circulating use alcohol as a preservative or absorption agent, including Releana. Although I initially used ethanol myself in sublingual mixing, and did lose weight, I was sharing the mix with a family member and mixed once a week. However, since then, according to the person in my group that is being treated by Dr B, he says that if sublingual is mixed with ethanol (drinking alcohol), it "melts" the hCG molecule chemically speaking, and degrades it significantly. Remember that alcohol is used in meat marinades to break down the protein so that it will be tender. Instead, colloidal silver is preferred because it does not seem to degrade the hCG and acts as an antiseptic to keep bacteria out of the mix. Why take a chance with drinking alcohol? My friend Shalom, who has videos on YouTube and you may have seen on the Mike and Juliet show, uses colloidal silver and B-12 to mix her sublingual recipe, and is having great weight reduction with her formula. You can see her mixing kits here: **http://tinyurl.com/SubMixKit**

General Steps for Mixing Sublingual hCG
1. Open appropriate solvent vial and hCG ampoule/vial as for injections.
2. Use a syringe to withdraw the appropriate solvent and inject it into the hCG ampoule.
3. It should dissolve quickly. DON'T SHAKE, but you can gently move or swirl the bottle around to assist it in dissolving.
4. After it's fully dissolved, withdraw it with the same syringe and inject it into the amber bottle.
5. Add the other ingredients into the amber bottle.

I believe that the following mix also could be used successfully:
1 ml appropriate solvent (same as what shipped with it) per every 1000 IU (10 ml for 10,000 IU)
1/10 ml sodium bicarbonate per every 1000 IU (1 ml for 10,000 IU) as a buffer (pH should be as close to 7.0 as possible, at least between 6.0 and 8.0.)
5/10 ml glycerin per every 1000 IU (5 ml glycerin for 10,000 IU)

This would produce a mix that would give about 666.66 IU per ml. Dividing that into two doses of 1/4 (.25) ml twelve hours apart per day, results in 333.33 IU per day.

Simplest Sublingual Mix Ever

Even the solvent alone, just as used for injections, has been successful for many as a sublingual mix. The simplest method is to mix 5,000 IU into 5 cc of the appropriate solvent and put into a sterile vial. 1,500 IU (1.5 cc) could be removed and mixed with additional appropriate solvent to dilute it to the dose per cc desired. For example, if 300 IU daily was desired, the 1,500 IU would make 5 doses. To use 0.25 cc twice a day, someone would mix it by adding 1 cc of appropriate solvent to the 1.5 cc hCG so that the total would be 2.5 cc (0.25 cc dose x 2 times a day x 5 doses).

In a small (10 or 15 ml) amber glass bottle, mix as follows:

For 1,500 IU:
4 ml of of Colloidal Silver
1 ml of sublingual B-12
1 1,500 IU ampoule of hCG

Use 1 cc of the Colloidal Silver part of your liquid to reconstitute your hCG, ensuring that you have a total of 5 ml of liquid with hCG mixed in when you're finished. If you take a 0.5 ml dose twice a day, it will give you a dosage of 300 IU per day for 7 days.

For 5,000 IU:
14 ml of Colloidal Silver
1 ml of sublingual B-12
5000 IU of hCG reconstituted with 1 cc of the Colloidal Silver

The above gives 333 IU per day, taking a 0.5 ml dose once in the morning and once in the evening (a total of 1 ml per day). The mixture is enough for 15 days. If you want to use a 7 day mixing cycle, just share half of it with a family member or friend.

Keep refrigerated. The key is to have a continuous amount of hCG in your system, so dosing is twice a day, 12 hours apart. Use the dropper or dosing syringe to withdraw the measured dose and squirt under your tongue. Hold the mixture under your tongue as long as possible, at least 5 minutes. Do not drink or eat for 15 minutes after dosing.

Homeopathic Dosing and Rules

Storage: No refrigeration required.
Dosing: 10 to 20 drops under the tongue 3x/day. No skipping of doses.
Some report better results with half the dose twice as often, though.
Wait 10 minutes prior to eating or drinking anything.
Do not use mint or caffeine while using homeopathic remedies.
If taking through the airport, do not send through x-ray; ask for manual inspection.
Only continue VLCD for 48 hours after last dose, not 72.

Storing hCG

The package inserts give storage temperatures for both the powdered hCG in the ampoule/vial and for mixed hCG. In general, the freeze-dried powder is fine at controlled room temperature 15° to 30° C (59° to 86° F). Once mixed, hCG is to be stored at 2° to 8° C (36° F to 46° F) in a refrigerator.

The following table shows the package insert information for various brands:

Brand	IU	Year	Excipients	Solvent	To Store	Storage Instructions / Claims
Hucog	2,000, 5,000, or 10,000IU	no date	Lactose or Mannitol I.P. Disodium hydrogen phosphate I.P. and Sodium dihydrogen phosphate I.P.	Sodium chloride 0.9%	Freeze-dried powder	Vials of HuCoG Inj. Should be stored at 2° – 8° C protected from light.
Pregnyl	1,500IU	2002 2005	Sodium carboxymethylcellulose 0.05 mg, Mannitol 5.0 mg, Disodium hydrogen phosphate, calculated as anhydrous 0.25 mg Sodium dihydrogen phosphate, calculated as anhydrous 0.25 mg.	Sodium chloride 0.9%	Unspecified	Special precautions for storage Store at 2 to 8°C. Do not freeze. Keep the ampoules in the outer container to protect from light. Discard any unused portion.
Provigil	1,000, 2,000, 5,000, 10,000IU	Unk	Mannitol I.P 12 mg, Potassium Dihydrogen Orthophosphate B.P.0.46 mg, and Dipotassium Hydrogen Orthophosphate B.P 0.36 mg	Sodium chloride 0.9%	Unspecified	Discard any unused portion.

Brand	IU	Year	Excipients	Solvent	To Store	Storage Instructions / Claims
Lupi	2,000, 5,000, or 10,000IU	Unk	Mannitol I.P 12 mg, Potassium Dihydrogen Orthophosphate B.P.0 46 mg, and Dipotassium Hydrogen Orthophosphate B.P 0.36 mg	Sodium chloride 0.9%	Unspecified	Discard any unused portion.
Pubergen	1,000, 2,000, 5,000 or 10,000IU	2007	Not Given	Sodium chloride 0.9%	Unspecified	To be stored under refrigeration between 8°C to 20°C. Do not freeze.
Profasi	2,000, 5,000, or 10,000IU	1993	Mannitol 100 mg, Dibasic Sodium Phosphate 16 mg, and Monobasic Sodium Phosphate 4 mg.	Bacteriostatic water with 0.9% benzyl alcohol	Freeze-dried powder	Store dry product at controlled room temperature 15°-30° C (59°-86° F).
					Reconstituted	AFTER RECONSTITUTION, REFRIGERATE THE PRODUCT AT 2°-8° C (36°-46° F) AND USE WITHIN 30 DAYS.
APP Abraxis	10,000IU	2008	Mannitol 100 mg, Monobasic sodium phosphate, Dibasic sodium phosphate	Bacteriostatic water with 0.9% benzyl alcohol	Unspecified	Store at 20° - 25° C (68° - 77° F) **IMPORTANT: USE COMPLETELY WITHIN 60 DAYS AFTER RECONSTITUTION. REFRIGERATE AFTER RECONSTITUTION.**
Novarel	10,000IU	2004	100 mg, Dibasic Sodium Phosphate 16 mg, and Monobasic Sodium Phosphate 4 mg.	Bacteriostatic water with 0.9% benzyl alcohol	Freeze-dried powder	The sterile lyophilized powder is stable. Store dry product at controlled room temperature 15° - 30° C (59° - 86° F).
					Reconstituted	To be stored under refrigeration between 8°C to 20°C. Do not freeze. When reconstituted with Bacteriostatic Water for Injection preserved with benzyl alcohol 0.9%, the solution should be refrigerated and used within 30 days.
A.P.L.	5,000 or 10,000IU	1974	Lactose: APL 5 000: 0.9%; APL 10 000: 1.8%.	2.0% Benzyl alcohol as a preservative, not more than 0.2% phenol	Freeze-dried powder	Store in a refrigerator, but do not freeze
					Reconstituted	After reconstitution, may be stored for 30 days in a refrigerator. Keep out of reach of children.
Pregnyl	10,000IU	1998	5 mg monobasic sodium phosphate and 4.4 mg dibasic sodium phosphate.	Sodium chloride 0.56% and benzyl alcohol 0.9%	Freeze-dried powder	Store at 15°–30°C (59°–86°F).
					Reconstituted	Reconstituted solution is stable for 60 days when refrigerated.

Brand	IU	Year	Excipients	Solvent	To Store	Storage Instructions / Claims
Pregnyl	10,000IU	2006	Monobasic sodium phosphate 5 mg, Dibasic sodium phosphate 4.4 mg	Sodium chloride 0.56% and benzyl alcohol 0.9%	Freeze-dried powder	Store at 15–30°C (59–86°F).
					Reconstituted	Reconstituted solution is stable for 60 days when refrigerated.
Pregnyl	1,500 or 5,000IU	1986	Not stated	Not stated	Unspecified	Store in a refrigerator between 2° - 8 °C. Protect from light. Keep out of reach of children.
Origen	Not Given	2007	Not Given	Not Given	Unspecified	To be stored under refrigeration between 8°C to 20°C. Do not freeze.

How long is mixed hCG potent?

Most hCG package inserts state 30 days if kept refrigerated. Some have been tested by bio-assay to be stable and active for 60 days. **http://tinyurl.com/Ninsert** **http://tinyurl.com/Pinsert**

However, probably the most reliable data would come from the ELISA standards for measuring free hCG used in controlled experiments. For storing hCG controls, the study designers state: "Reconstituted [hCG] standards should be stored sealed at 2° to 8° C (36° F to 46° F) and it will be stable for at least two weeks at that condition." Since these are controls, they have to have stable hCG levels, so we know it's good at least 14 days in a cool, dry place, probably in the refrigerator.

Mixed hCG is stored in a sterile sealed glass vial (amber is preferred to block the light) because elements DO affect the potency. Air exposure, light exposure, heat, and extreme cold (freezing) will damage the structure of the proteins in the hCG. Some clinics do pre-fill syringes for convenience. If you can, draw out your dosage just before you are ready for injection to minimize exposure to air and light. Storing prefilled syringes in the refrigerator has worked well for me. It takes about an hour to get them all filled if you are mixing with 5000 IU. You can test your hCG solution by putting some drops of it on a pregnancy test to see if it is hCG, but it does not tell you HOW active it still is, only that it is real hCG and that it is active enough to register on the test.

Can hCG be frozen to prolong its potency?

hCG cannot be frozen. It states this specifically on the Pregnyl package insert. The Novarel brand and other brand's inserts do not include freezing temperatures in the storage instructions. Freezing can damage the protein. When a protein such as hCG is frozen or heated, the bonds are broken that hold the protein's shape, which disrupts the structure of the molecule, which causes the protein to become biologically inactive. One of my support group members learned this fact in pre-nursing courses. It was also brought up again in her pharmacology course in reference to insulin (which is also a large molecule hormone and a protein just as hCG is) and storage of it. It was taught that if it were frozen, it would need to be thrown away and a new vial that had not been frozen would need to be used. Once you freeze a protein, it's no longer viable. I have confirmed this information with both a doctor and a pharmacist. Since hCG is a hormone with a specific molecular structure, freezing would fracture this structure and make it inactive. Another support group member had two separate stalls of more than 5 days because of frozen hCG, so I wouldn't chance it. I know that various companies and clinics that provide hCG instruct customers to freeze their pre-filled syringes and then thaw them for use, but this is in direct contradiction to the storage instructions for the drug. If you do decide to freeze your hCG syringes, it is important not to thaw them at room temperature. Put them in the refrigerator to thaw.

Freezing protein is a very tricky business: **http://tinyurl.com/freezingprotein**
http://tinyurl.com/freezingprotein2

If you are at all concerned about how long the hCG will last in the fridge, then here is a suggestion. After injecting on day 23, throw out the remaining mixed hCG and mix a new batch the next morning for the remaining days. This way each batch is only in the fridge for 23 days maximum. Since you are going to be using both ampoules or vials anyway, and then throwing out what is left over at the end, this is a way to ensure potency.

Safety Tips for discarding syringes and needles

Consider using self-sheathing needles for your protection and others. *DO NOT REUSE NEEDLES.* Needles should be disposed of in a safe manner. Puncture resistant containers, called Sharps containers, can be purchased online, through medical supply stores, and some pharmacies, including Costco.

Some cities offer free Sharps containers/disposal at certain centers. Check with your city on proper disposal. If Sharps containers are unavailable, place used needles in a thick container such as a plastic drink bottle or a liquid laundry detergent container, seal with a lid, label as a bio-hazard, and discard in the trash. **NEVER discard syringes with needles directly in the trash, as the needle cap could come off and cause a waste collector concern and an unnecessary HIV test.**

Step 29 – Begin your hCG administration method of choice.

Injecting hCG

If your clinic or physician has sent you home with pre-mixed hCG for your weight reduction protocol, these tips may help with self-administration of your hCG shots. Most of us were nervous about self-injecting. And we all got over it once we did the first shot. It's far easier than we thought and most comment "It didn't hurt at all," or "I didn't even feel it."

What helped me was doing the EFT tapping for it since EFT works for phobias very well. Try **http://tinyurl.com/EFTmanual** or search EFT on YouTube for videos that you can follow along with. It will decrease your anxiety tremendously! It takes only 5 minutes to learn it and use it for your needle/injection phobia and it was well worth the time. Looks stupid, works great!

Self-injection tips can also be found in the following illustrations and videos:

SC Illustrations
http://tinyurl.com/SCInj
http://tinyurl.com/SCInj2

Videos
SC: **http://tinyurl.com/SCInjVid**
SC: **http://tinyurl.com/SCInjVid2**
IM: **http://tinyurl.com/IMInjVid**
IM: **http://tinyurl.com/IMInjVid2**

Reading the Measurement on the Syringe

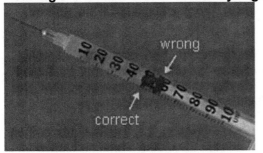

I wasn't sure how to read the measurements on a syringe and this photo helped. You read from the line closest to the pointed end of the plunger. Pay no attention to the .5 cc (ml) dosage being measured in the photo, since you will most likely be injecting 1 cc (ml).

Try to minimize the time that the finished solution is left out at room temperature. When you prepare your daily injection, fill your syringe and replace the hCG vial back in the refrigerator quickly. Alcohol wipes are necessary for cleaning the top of the vials, the ampoules, and to clean the injection site.

The vial has a vacuum in it. You need to put as much air into the vial as the amount of liquid you want to draw out:
1. Pull back on the plunger to whatever dosage you are planning on using
2. Turn the glass vial of hCG upside down
3. Insert the needle into the center of the rubber top of the vial
4. Inject the air into the glass vial
5. Keep the vial upside down while you withdraw the solution
6. Draw out a bit more than what you need and then inject the excess back into the vial before withdrawing the needle
7. Do not touch the needle
8. Put the cap back on the needle
9. Let your dose warm up to room temperature

It is recommended that you change the needle after you draw out your daily injection from the hCG vial. This is due to the fact that the needle will dull up to 50% when it pierces through the hard rubber top of the vial. A new SHARP needle will cause you less pain when injecting.

Before switching needles:
o Draw back a tiny bit to draw the solution out of the needle
o Remove that needle while keeping the syringe tip pointed up
o Pull back on the plunger to bring more air into the syringe
o Flick the syringe while pointing the needle end at the ceiling to remove any bubbles or air
o Push out all the excess air
o Put on a new needle to use for injecting

Easing the discomfort of hCG injections

For less pain, allow medications that have been refrigerated to warm to room temperature before injection. It helps to put the filled syringe under your arm for about five minutes to warm it more quickly. If you are too busy flailing around trying to get ready for work, and your armpit is not a safe place to warm the syringe, place the cap back on the needle to keep it sterile, and then rest the syringe on top of your warm coffee/tea cup and hop in the shower. When you get out of the shower, the hCG is a perfect temperature.

Clean the selected injection area with an alcohol swab in a circular motion, from center out. Allowing the alcohol to air dry before injecting will somewhat ease the discomfort of the shot so that it will sting less. Pinching the skin and pulling it out gently can also provide distraction to your nerves so that you do not feel the needle. You can also apply ice to numb the location prior to injection.

Relaxing the muscles also reduces pain. Relax the muscles prior to injection. It is true that this is often difficult when injecting yourself because we tend to tense up. To relax the glutes, stand and put most of your weight on the opposite leg in a relaxed tip-toe stance or bend your leg slightly on the side where you are injecting. For the arm, hold it at a 90 degree angle. If you are injecting into your thigh, be sitting down.

Injecting procedure
1. Select a site and cleanse the area (about 2 inches) with a fresh alcohol pad, or cotton ball soaked in alcohol.
2. Wait for the site to dry.
3. Remove the needle cap.
4. Check for an air bubble. Point the needle straight up and flick the syringe with your finger to move any air bubbles to the top, and then slowly depress the plunger to remove any air. You will see the air travel up and then see a drop of solution form at the tip of the needle.
5. Hold the syringe the way you would a pencil or dart. Some people prefer the quick motion shot, while others prefer resting the needle on the pinched skin and pushing it through in a smooth motion. You do not need to insert the entire needle if you can reach muscle without doing so when doing IM. Insert the needle at a 90 degree angle for IM (using a longer needle) or 45 degree if SC. If you are doing it IM, then inject at 90 degrees to the skin (and either use a shorter needle or don't insert it as far).
6. Aspiration: Hold the syringe with one hand. With the other, pull back the plunger very slightly to check for blood. If you see blood in the solution in the syringe, do not inject. Withdraw the needle and start again at a new site with a "new" needle—change the needle. If you do not see blood, slowly push the plunger to inject the medication. Press the plunger all the way down. Inject the medication quickly or slowly, whichever is more comfortable for you.
7. Remove the needle from the skin and gently hold an alcohol pad on the injection site. Do not rub. It is not abnormal to see a small amount of bleeding at the injection site. Direct pressure with your finger or a cotton ball or swab will stop the bleeding and prevent bruising of the skin. Hitting little capillaries is easy to do and there are no side effects. If you bleed or bruise after the injection, that is usually because you pierced a very small blood vessel with the needle on the way to the muscle. It doesn't mean the tip of the needle was in the blood vessel when you injected. If you pull back on the plunger and no blood returns in the syringe, you are not in a blood vessel. Slight swelling, redness, burning, or itching is not uncommon and should subside shortly.
8. Immediately cap the needle and put the syringe/needle into the disposal container.

If you forget the aspiration step and put it in the vein by accident, it would be metabolized faster, and so maybe you wouldn't have a longer term (24-hour) effect. (This is the main reason you should make sure you are not in a vein by aspirating for blood.) Second, IF you are in a vein, and you inject a WHOLE LOT of air (not just the tiny specks of bubbles, but multiple ccs of air), then the air in the vein could cause a problem in the heart. Finally, if you are unlucky enough to have a ventral septal defect in the heart (hole between the two bottom chambers) and inject air into a vein by accident, even in smaller amounts such as one whole cc of air, then it could go straight to the arterial system and to the brain, causing possible injury to the brain.

I'm not saying that you should ever intentionally inject air into your veins, but your body can absorb quite a bit. In fact, **www.emedicine.com** states that more than 5 ml per kg is needed to cause significant complications, although it states that as little as 20 ml (around the amount of air in an unprimed IV line) has been reported to cause some problems. Large amounts (of between 100 to 300 ml) have allegedly been fatal.

I listed all of the very worst, very unlikely, possibilities. It's hard to even imagine a scenario in which you would have an accidental serious injury if you didn't aspirate and check for blood in the syringe (there's no way that you are going to be injecting a whole cc of air), but you do want to make sure the hCG goes where you intend so that you get the effect that you want, based on the rate of absorption.

Rotating Injection Sites

It is very important to rotate injection sites, to avoid cellulitis (**http://tinyurl.com/cellulitisinfo**) or abscesses (**http://tinyurl.com/abscessinfo**). Do not use the same site for injections each time. Rotate your injection sites in a regular pattern. You should be at least 1 ½ inches away from the last injection site. Jot down on your calendar where you gave your last shot. This will help prevent giving the shot in the same place too soon.

Subcutaneous Injections

SC syringes can be as small as 1 or ½ cc (ml). Needles are 29 to 33 gauge. Needle angle should be 45 degrees, to inject into fat rather than muscle.

Intramuscular Injections

The IM syringe size needed is 3 cc (ml). Some people have reported less stinging with IM when using 25 or 27 gauge than with 30 gauge needles.

Needle angle should be 90 degrees, (straight in). Otherwise it is likely to enter subcutaneous tissues instead. (Length of the needle is chosen based on the amount of subcutaneous tissue that must be penetrated to reach muscle.)

A 1 ½" needle for the arm or leg is quite long unless you have a good bit of subcutaneous tissue (fat) in that area. To check, pinch the fat on the front of the leg and arm (not the back of the arm, the side of the arm, deltoid muscle) to see how much you have. If you can easily feel muscle, use a 1" needle, if you can pinch an inch or more of tissue and cannot feel muscle, then the longer needle is okay. You don't want to hit bone or blood vessels. Also, you don't have to insert the needle all the way to the hub of the needle. (For those that don't know what the hub is, it's where the needle meets the syringe). Stomach muscles are too thin (even in most muscle builders), calves may be large, but the normal paths of blood vessels and nerves are unpredictable. Use only the following sites for IM.

Vastus lateralis site

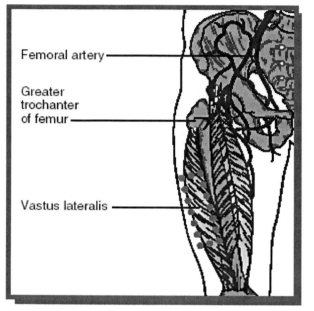

Femoral artery

Greater trochanter of femur

Vastus lateralis

The outer thigh is the spot most often used for self administered injections. Notice that the target muscle is at the outside of either thigh, midway between knee and top of thigh. Injecting in the top of the thigh could hit nerve, major blood vessel, or bone.

Deltoid site

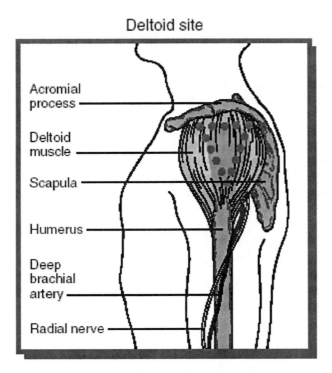

Acromial
process

Deltoid
muscle

Scapula

Humerus

Deep
brachial
artery

Radial nerve

Deltoid site in upper arm is a
triangle shaped area of muscle.
This site is hard to use on
yourself but one of the safest if
someone gives the shot to you.
Also, usually allows the smallest
(shortest) needle.

Dorsogluteal site

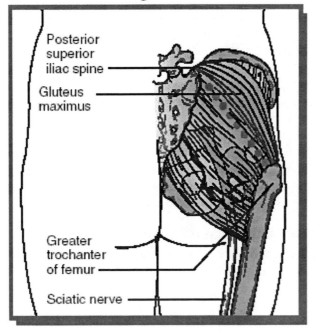

Posterior
superior
iliac spine

Gluteus
maximus

Greater
trochanter
of femur

Sciatic nerve

Upper outer quadrant of the gluteus
maximus muscle is the largest
muscle, so least likely to hit a nerve.
But there is a very important nerve,
(sciatic), running through it. So be
sure to aim below the hip bone but
still high and to the side of the hip.
Shots in the hip should NOT be in
the middle of the hip. Difficult for self-
injecting.

Step 30 –Decide how to handle other people while on the diet.

I want to do this, but my significant other disagrees. What can I do?

You are ultimately the one responsible for your own health and what you do concerning your own body. A true partner in love will understand and honor that. Sometimes, it is difficult for a partner to recognize your autonomy, especially if he/she fears for your well-being. Taking the time to show your partner the research in this book, especially the links, can help him/her to let go and trust that you are capable of looking out for your own best interests. Remind your partner that remaining overweight or obese is a health risk that you already bear and that this protocol has the potential to remove that risk from your life for good. Ask him/her not to make this process more difficult for you by opposing you and instead, request that he/she provide you the partnering, encouragement, love, and support that can be so critical for someone beginning a transformational adventure such as this. You might want to put all of this in a sweet loving letter.

What should I tell people who ask me what I am doing?

This diet can be difficult for others to understand because they have not done the research and verified for themselves that it is safe and effective. You may wish to avoid discussing it until your obvious weight reduction success and good health are undeniable. One way to do this is to explain that you are following a plan designed by a medical doctor who researched it for many years, which is true.

I heard that one person is using the creative and humorous reply that he was having alien liposuction during abduction experiences every night. That seems guaranteed to change the subject…!

Step 31 – Weigh yourself each day and record the weight in the Pounds and Inches Tracking Spreadsheet.

Weigh yourself each day and record the weight in the Pounds and Inches Tracking Spreadsheet.

How do I calculate the average daily weight reduction?

Dr. S says that the average reduction of weight is calculated on the number of effective injections and therefore we use the weight reached on the day of the third injection which may be well above what it was 2 days earlier when the first injection was given. That is your weight on the first VLCD day of 500 calories after the load days.

Step 32 – Load TO CAPACITY with lots of fats for the first two days of hCG.

Load TO CAPACITY with lots of fats for the first two days of hCG administration. Examples: black olives, macadamia nuts, walnuts, avocados, Italian sausage, bacon, braunschweiger or liverwurst, heavy cream, sour cream, cheese, whipping cream, butter, coconut oil, and cream cheese.

Do I have to load/gorge the first two days of hCG administration?

YES! Otherwise, you risk serious hunger problems during the first week of VLCD. Eat LOTS of FAT, rather than lots of sugar, though. Don't worry; the load weight will come off very quickly, usually within 48 hours.

Step 33 – Begin the 500 calorie food plan (VLCD) on day three.

What does VLCD mean?
Very Low Calorie Diet, which is 500 calories.

Isn't 500 calories a day unhealthy?
Page 63 of Pounds and Inches states, "Just as the daily dose of HCG is the same in all cases, so the same diet proves to be satisfactory for a small elderly lady of leisure or a hard working muscular giant. Under the effect of HCG the obese body is always able to obtain all the Calories it needs from the abnormal fat deposits, regardless of whether it uses up 1500 or 4000 per day. It must be made very clear to the patient that he is living to a far greater extent on the fat which he is losing than on what he eats."

This is reinforced again on page 65, "Sooner or later most patients express a fear that they may be running out of vitamins or that the restricted diet may make them anemic. On this score the physician can confidently relieve their apprehension by explaining that every time they lose a pound of fatty tissue, which they do almost daily, only the actual fat is burned up; all the vitamins, the proteins, the blood, and the minerals which this tissue contains in abundance are fed back into the body. Actually, a low blood count not due to any serious disorder of the blood forming tissues improves during treatment, and we have never encountered a significant protein deficiency nor signs of a lack of vitamins in patients who are dieting regularly."

And again on page 103, "Thus when we speak of a 500 Calorie diet this means that the body is being supplied with as much fuel as would be required to raise the temperature of 500 liters of water by 1 degree Centigrade or 50 liters by 10 degrees. This is quite insufficient to cover the heat and energy requirements of an adult body. In the HCG method the deficit is made up from the abnormal fat-deposits, of which **1 lb. furnishes the body with more than 2000 Calories**. As this is roughly the amount lost every day, a patient under HCG is never short of fuel."

Can't I eat more than 500 calories and still lose?
Dr S states on page 49, "Even seemingly insignificant deviations, particularly those that at first sight seem to be an improvement, are very liable to produce most disappointing results and even annul the effect completely. For instance, if the diet is increased from 500 to 600 or 700 Calories, the loss of weight is quite unsatisfactory."

Won't anyone lose weight on 500 calories a day, without hCG?
Here are some reasons why a 500 calorie diet without hCG is NOT the way to go:
  o Without hCG, you will be extremely hungry because your body will be starving for nutrients. Dr S tells us that hCG causes over 2000 calories to be released from your abnormal fat stores into your bloodstream daily, so although you are eating 500 calories, your nutritional needs are served by the total calories in your bloodstream.
  o Without this effect, your basal metabolism would become even slower, causing you to gain weight the minute that you resume normal eating.
  o Because your body will be starving without hCG, it will attempt to store everything you eat as fat.

If you take the time to research the effects of a 500 calorie diet without hCG, I believe you will find that attempting a VLCD without hCG can harm your health, possibly permanently.

Do I have to eat all 500 calories each day?

According to Dr. Simeons on page 61, "Those not uncommon patients who feel that even so little food is too much for them, can omit anything they wish." That having been said, some people have reported better results when eating the entire 500 calories, especially the vegetables allowed each day, rather than omitting them. One person kept waiting for the burst-of-energy feeling that everyone says they get from the injections. It hadn't happened. As a matter of fact, she felt awful. She was very weak and tired all the time. She found out after a trip to the doctor and blood tests why she felt so awful. She hadn't been eating enough and had made herself anemic. I don't think that Dr. Simeons meant to omit entire meals, two days at a time, nor to omit the protein, since he states that we are on the verge of protein deficiency. Some of us have discovered that if we eat less than 400 calories, we won't lose, but if we eat more than 500 calories, we won't lose. The sweet spot is in the 400 to 500 calories range.

I got sick while on the diet and wasn't able to eat, so I didn't lose. What do I do now?

The not eating at all while sick might have thrown you into starvation mode. If it were me, I'd try an all protein day of 500 calories of all protein to get going again.

I just found out that I have to have surgery soon. Do I have to stop the diet?

I personally would not continue 500 calories right just to ensure that my body had everything needed to heal the surgical wound properly, but that's just me. Yes, we are releasing nutrients stored in fat, but what if what I burned off that day didn't happen to have all the vitamins, protein, and especially vitamin C that my body needed that day to heal after the surgery?

How much water is optimal for this weight reduction protocol?

I tested this on two people. Both noticed a weight reduction rate increase when they cut down from drinking a gallon of water a day to between 2 and 2.5 liters a day. Dr S said at least 2 liters. Here is a mantra: "If you drink enough, you shrink enough." You will need to up the intake if you are in a warmer climate or are exercising. Don't worry, you won't run to the bathroom every twenty minutes after your body adjusts to the higher level of fluid intake.

Sweeteners

On page 63 of the original text, Dr. S says "In many countries specially prepared and low calorie foods are freely available and some of these can be tentatively used."

In fact, when the first support group for refined carbohydrate addiction was formed, it was believed that saccharin did not cause a reaction like refined carbohydrates did. Specifically, it was believed that it did not trigger the pancreas to release insulin because saccharin does not convert to glucose in the bloodstream. However, this study showed that saccharin did indeed trigger insulin release: **http://tinyurl.com/SaccharinInsulin**

You can also view Sweet Misery online here: **http://tinyurl.com/SweetMis**

Xylitol is a sugar alcohol, like maltitol, mannitol, etc. I would think that it would be self-limiting, in that it will give you loose stools if overused. However, I would not use it for Phase 2, because it is not zero calorie, only low-glycemic. Erythritol is a better choice in that it is the only sugar alcohol that doesn't have the digestive side-effect with overuse and it is closest to zero-calorie. I think that pure stevia without any fillers is better, but you could try it and see, although I wouldn't overdo it. The new stevia sweetener Truvia does contain erythritol as a filler.

So what SHOULD we use for a sweetener?

I use only Stevia as a sweetener-- it will really benefit you to give up Splenda, Aspartame, and MSG (in their many forms and hidden names on the label). They all make you hungrier and fuel addictions, not to mention other terrible effects: **http://tinyurl.com/excitotoxins**

In a recent study by Duke University, rats that were fed Splenda (sucralose) for only three months gained 9%-12% more weight than those that were not. Even more frightening, those rats continued to gain more after the Splenda was discontinued. "Splenda Alters Gut Microflora and Increases Intestinal P-Glycoprotein and Cytochrome P-450 in Male Rats" Journal of Toxicology and Environmental Health Part A, vol. 71, No. 21, January 2008 **http://tinyurl.com/DukeStudy**

I am often asked about the Walden Farms products and if they can be used on this diet. For me, Walden Farms would fall into the category of "fake food" that I don't want in my diet anymore. A theory exists that if you ingest stuff that your body doesn't recognize; it tags it as a toxin and stores it in fat. Sometimes extra fat must be created and stored in order to do this. I would rather eat real food that my body knows how to eliminate. For example, studies show that only 70-80% of Splenda is excreted. Wonder where the rest goes? Although Splenda in particular is not fat soluble and would not be stored in fat, I believe that the body might sequester other fake chemical ingredients in WF products in fat, which if you don't have enough of, it would be forced to create more fat in order to protect you from the perceived toxin. And I have to wonder if the metabolites of Splenda that represent the 20-30% that was absorbed into the body are really what I want as the building blocks for my cells?

Truvia (from Coke-Cargill) or PureVia (from Pepsi-Merisant) might work on P2 if the erythritol included with the stevia does not stall you. Although I prefer the brands such as SweetLeaf, and trust their extraction methods more than I do the larger companies' methods, this sweetener is probably much better for you than aspartame, sucralose, or saccharin. Diet sodas will be available soon from the big soda manufacturers with Truvia and PureVia as the sweetener. Sobe LifeWater already has a delicious 0 cal version with PureVia. I have tried the Zevia diet colas with Stevia. Not bad at all. I avoid drinking much soda, though, even with stevia. The high phosphoric acid is unhealthy.

Safety of Stevia

Scientists who have studied Stevia state that it is safe for human consumption. It is even safe for diabetics. Stevia is a dietary supplement that is "0" on the glycemic index because it contains fiber and is suitable for all people, including diabetics.

Here's the most recent research to answer the question, "Is stevia toxic?" According to a study published in 2003 in the *Phytochemistry* journal, "Acute and subacute toxicity studies revealed a very low toxicity of Stevia and stevioside." Read the abstract for yourself at PubMed: **http://tinyurl.com/steviastudy**.

Stevia Cooking Conversion Chart:
http://tinyurl.com/SteviaConv

Can I keep taking my vitamins or supplements during the diet?

Dr. Simeons addresses taking vitamins in his book. He writes on page 65 that there are enough stored in our fat cells to sustain us as they are released during fat reduction:
"Vitamins and anemia
Sooner or later most patients express a fear that they may be running out of vitamins or that the

restricted diet may make them anemic. On this score the physician can confidently relieve their apprehension by explaining that every time they lose a pound of fatty tissue, which they do almost daily, only the actual fat is burned up; all the vitamins, the proteins, the blood, and the minerals which this tissue contains in abundance are fed back into the body. Actually, a low blood count not due to any serious disorder of the blood forming tissues improves during treatment, and we have never encountered a significant protein deficiency nor signs of a lack of vitamins in patients who are dieting regularly."

That being said, if the fat that you are releasing was stored when you were not eating healthily, you might not get all the nutrients you need when it is released. I would not take vitamins with oils.

Can I continue to take my medications?

I would consult with my health care practitioner before discontinuing any medication. In my support group, people have had success either way. Simeons did allow thyroid medication when the thyroid had been completely or partially removed.

Can I take birth control pills while doing the hCG injections?

Dr. Simeons states that oral contraceptives may be used during treatment. IUDs should be fine.

Should I be concerned about drug testing for a job interview, or standard bloodwork at my checkup, if I am taking hCG at the time?

Job interview drug testing, unless it includes a pregnancy test, and it shouldn't, won't show the hCG is in your system.

Although it is certainly no cause for alarm, **http://tinyurl.com/cholester** your yearly physical could show higher than normal Cholesterol levels while you are taking hCG, according to Dr S:
"Cholesterol
The exact extent to which the blood cholesterol is involved in hardening of the arteries, high blood pressure and coronary disease is not as yet known, but it is now widely admitted that the blood cholesterol level is governed by diencephalic mechanisms. The behavior of circulating cholesterol is therefore of particular interest during the treatment of obesity with HCG.

Cholesterol circulates in two forms, which we call free and esterified. Normally these fractions are present in a proportion of about 25% free to 75% esterified cholesterol, and it is the latter fraction which damages the walls of the arteries. In pregnancy this proportion is reversed and it may he taken for granted that arteriosclerosis never gets worse during pregnancy for this very reason.

To my knowledge, the only other condition in which the proportion of free to esterified cholesterol is reversed is during the treatment of obesity with HCG + diet, when exactly the same phenomenon takes place. This seems an important indication of how closely a patient under HCG treatment resembles a pregnant woman in diencephalic behavior.

When the total amount of circulating cholesterol is normal before treatment, this absolute amount is neither significantly increased nor decreased. But when an obese patient with an abnormally high cholesterol and already showing signs of arteriosclerosis is treated with HCG, his blood pressure drops and his coronary circulation seems to improve, and yet his total blood cholesterol may soar to heights never before reached.

At first this greatly alarmed us. But then we saw that the patients came to no harm even if treatment was continued and we found in follow-up examinations undertaken some months after treatment that the cholesterol was much better than it had been before treatment. As the increase is mostly in the form of the not dangerous free cholesterol, we gradually came to welcome the phenomenon. Today we believe that the rise is entirely due to the liberation of recent cholesterol deposits that have not yet undergone calcification in the arterial wall and therefore highly beneficial."

Don't I need to exercise to lose weight?

Some people have reported that they get better results with exercising, but Dr. Simeons does not state that it is necessary. Nor do clinical studies suggest that exercise causes weight reduction: **http://tinyurl.com/TaubesExercise** Many members have reported satisfactory weight reduction without it. One hCG clinic actually asks that patients wait until they are down to within 10 or 20 pounds of their goal weight before beginning any impact or strenuous exercise: **http://tinyurl.com/hcgclinic**

Along with being misled about diet, we have been sold a bill of goods when it comes to the best ways to exercise, too. Aerobic exercise (cardio) actually ensures that your heart and lungs have no reserves. When you do return to exercise, I recommend the program developed by Al Sears, MD instead: **http://tinyurl.com/AlSearsMD**.

Can I use exercise to burn off some calories that I shouldn't have eaten?

"Calories in, calories out" is a lie in my opinion. The research that I have seen shows that the KIND of calorie is important, the mix of fat, carbs, and protein that is eaten determines whether or not fat is stored, and the experiences of my support group bears it out, that in particular, with the hCG Diet, it just doesn't work to try to offset a "cheat" with exercise.

Women only: How will my period affect this diet?

Some clinics advise continuing hCG during the menses and many have done so without problems. You may not lose during this time, however.

Here is exactly what Dr. Simeons says:
"Starting treatment
In menstruating women, the best time to start treatment is immediately after a period. Treatment may also be started later, but it is advisable to have at least ten days in hand before the onset of the next period. Similarly, the end of a course should never be made to coincide with onset of menstruation. If things should happen to work out that way, it is better to give the last injection three days before the expected date of the menses so that a normal diet can be resumed at onset. Alternatively, at least three injections should be given after the period, followed by the usual three days of dieting. This rule need not be observed in such patients who have reached their normal weight before the end of treatment and are already on a higher caloric diet." p. 59

Here is another section where he addresses stopping the hCG when you get your period:
"Menstruation
During menstruation no injections are given, but the diet is continued and causes no hardship; yet as soon as the menstruation is over, the patients become extremely hungry unless the injections are resumed at once. It is very impressive to see the suffering of a woman who has continued her diet for a day or two beyond the end of the period without coming for her injection and then to hear the next day that all hunger ceased within a few hours after the injection and to see her once again content, florid and cheerful." p. 54

Do I have to stop the hCG injections while I am menstruating?

It is a personal decision. Dr. Simeons states to do so, presumably to prevent a heavier flow. Many group members have not done so, with no ill effects.

My fat is getting soft and flabby where it used to be tight. ???

We have all seen this. It is the fat being mobilized for removal. You will notice it feels and looks different, squishy, jiggly, sort of. It's a GOOD THING, and it goes away once you discontinue the hCG.

What if I have to stop the protocol unexpectedly?

In Dr. Simeons' book on page 79, he says that if you have to go away or be social for a few days, you should stop hCG 3 days before you go away so that you can do 72 hours of VLCD after your last dose, but that if you have not had at least 20 days with both hCG and VLCD, you are more likely to regain the weight.

What if I need to travel during the diet?

I'll let my support group members answer this one:

"I've traveled and easily took my hCG with me. The first time, I stopped at a store and bought a large cup of ice and kept my needles in it. Another time, I had an empty shoe box in the car and put a Wal-Mart sack inside it, poured ice in it, and laid my needles inside. I've since purchased a small ice chest. It was easy for me to stay on the diet while traveling. I bought one of the little plastic bottles in the cosmetic department at Wal-Mart and filled it about half full of AVC (apple cider vinegar with "mother") and carried it in my purse."

"I would mail (overnight or 2nd day air) it ahead to the hotel (or wherever) and mix it when you get there. This is where a 1500 IU ampoule will come in handy. Just make arrangements for them to hold your package at the desk until you arrive."

"I also travel quite frequently and have had no issues traveling with either the hCG injectable or Releana. I simply take a small insulated bag with two gel packs (hard plastic) and ask the TSA agent to hand check the items. They have not asked for a prescription, only once did I get any objection from the agent and that was in objection to the hand check, said it wasn't a prescription so why did I want it hand checked (Releana did not look like a prescription) . After a brief explanation, I didn't want my medications to go through the x-ray machine, I had checked all the rules and this was a valid request, he went ahead and hand checked the items for me. As for the syringe, you are supposed to have a prescription to carry them on a plane; I simply put them in my checked luggage."

Take your weight reduction on the road with you with Joy Mangano's ingenious Fold-A-Weigh Scale. The sleek silver tone scale with a textured non-slip surface folds in half for easy packing or storage. At approximately 2 lbs and the size of a video cassette, your scale can go anywhere with you. Use your new scale as a weight reduction journal. Not only does it tell you your current weight, it tracks the target and previous 10 weights for up to 5 people.

Why do I feel so much better while on hCG?

Commercial preparations of hCG contain beta-endorphin. This neuropeptide has been demonstrated to affect the function of limbic-emotional circuits. Therefore, the beta-endorphin fraction present in commercial preparations of hCG could account for the mood control activity.

Step 34 – Record your food each day.

Record your food each day, to be used for analysis purposes later, if not reducing weight.

Help! What do I do about hunger during the first few days on hCG?

My first round of Phase 2 I was hungry the first week. I am now in my second round of Phase 2 and I am RARELY hungry. What is the difference between the two rounds? The only thing I can think of is that I did a yeast cleanse between rounds one and two which I did not do before starting this diet.

Another factor might have been that I did not eat a lot of fats on my two-day gorgefest, but instead had a lot of sugar and starch. Big mistake! Eat FAT on your loading days to avoid the experience that I had the first time, which seemed like a brush with starvation at first.

It lasted about a week and I had to do some real soul-searching. But I'm glad I did. If you're not writing in a diet journal every day, try it. It may help you understand why you want to eat even though you're not hungry and you've been SO SUCCESSFUL on this diet. During that week, I learned about food's role in my life up to that point and had to assign it a different, more minor role. I encourage you to stick through this tough period. This is a time to learn something and grow, if you take advantage of it.

On my second round, I looked up a list of high-fat foods to eat while loading: black olives, macadamia nuts, walnuts, avocados, Italian sausage, bacon, braunschweiger or liverwurst, heavy cream, sour cream, cheese, whipping cream, butter, coconut oil, and cream cheese.

One other factor that could come into play: If you are doing subcutaneous injections or even if you think you are doing IM injections, but you are using a needle shorter than 1" and could in reality be getting SC instead, you may not have built up a sufficient hCG level to really start mobilizing the abnormal fats for energy yet. Subcutaneous absorption is slower. The original plan assumes it takes two days to build up hCG levels doing IM injection, so that you can start your VLCD. If you are doing subcutaneous, it could take more than two days.

Also, your body can tell you that you are hungry when in fact, you are not. The sight or smell of nearby food is one of those things that can induce the insulin secretion that makes us think we're hungry. Or you could be mistaking thirst for hunger. Try drinking some water or a hot beverage such as tea.

Are you using powdered Stevia that has maltodextrin in it? Change to liquid Stevia, a brand that does not contain alcohol.

The other thing I've fought with is "empty stomach" vs. actual hunger. There are times I think I'm hungry, but my tummy is just completely empty.

One recipe is helpful to not feel as hungry:
100 grams of chicken breast or lean beef
½ a small head of cabbage cut into bite sized pieces (substitute spinach if cabbage stalls you, as it does me)
1 - 2 tablespoons of apple cider vinegar with the "mother"
1 tsp minced garlic
salt and pepper

Stir fry the meat dry over medium heat, stirring frequently to keep it from burning because there is NO oil used. If the meat starts to stick, add a small amount of water. Add cabbage and all other ingredients. Then stir frequently until cabbage is soft. Now, this isn't a deviation from the diet and it will make you feel FULL. It was the only thing that made me feel satisfied during that week. You could also do this with beef and add spices like onion, tomatoes (count it as a fruit), and chili powder and cayenne pepper for chili.

On this protocol, you cannot afford to let yourself get hungry. I have only cheated when I have not planned ahead and had the right food available when I needed it. For some reason, drinking the Yerba Mate tea or other hot drinks during the day and an ACV cocktail (glass of water with some Apple Cider Vinegar and a little liquid Stevia if you can't take the tartness) at night when I feel hungry really helps me.

Where can I find more information on the Callahan technique / EFT to help me with cravings or needle phobia?

A free manual is available at: **http://tinyurl.com/EFTmanual**

Help! I released 10 pounds the first week, but now I'm not reducing by 1 pound every day anymore. What am I doing wrong?

Absolutely Nothing. Dr. S states on page p. 51 "...the duration of treatment can be roughly assessed on the basis of an average loss of weight of a little less than a pound, say 300-400 grams - per injection, per day. It is a particularly interesting feature of the HCG treatment that in reasonably cooperative patients this figure is remarkably constant, regardless of sex, age and degree of overweight." And on page 67, "There may be no drop at all for two or three days and then a sudden loss which reestablishes the normal average. These fluctuations are entirely due to variations in the retention and elimination of water, which are more marked in women than in men." And again on page 68 "A plateau always corrects, itself, but many patients who have become accustomed to a regular daily loss get unnecessarily worried and begin to fret."

I learned everything that I needed to know about stalls in nursery school. "You get what you get and you don't get upset." Please quit panicking over something that is to be expected. Relax! Some of the possible reasons for this are explained in the next section.

What can I take for constipation?

For those who want to do something to produce a BM instead of just waiting for it to eventually happen on its own, try a laxative tea that contains cascara sagrada (instead of senna, which is harsh and can be addicting, causing you to become dependent), magnesium, digestive enzymes, vitamin C, or a tablespoon of coconut oil.

If all else fails, try glycerin suppositories, which work very quickly so make sure you are near a toilet. Also, for some, the detox bath at night with Epsom salt and baking soda will do the trick the next morning.

However, if you are eating only 500 calories a day, Dr. S says that you will only need to have a BM every 4 or 5 days (Simeons, p. 72). When you start to worry and your weight isn't dropping like normal, be sure you actually need to go. In other words do you feel the pressure to go or is it that you think it's time you need to do something about it?

What if I think that I am retaining water, with swollen ankles and fingers?

Drink Cornsilk tea for water retention in Phase 2. For Phase 3 water retention (hunger-edema caused by protein deficiency), eat two eggs for breakfast, a huge steak at lunch, and another huge steak plus a large helping of cheese for dinner to bring your protein level higher for that day and then continue P3, but with more protein than you were eating.

My hair has started to fall out. ???

Off the top of my head (excuse the pun), hair loss can be triggered by pregnancy or any stressful event such as the rapid weight reduction that occurs on this diet. It peaks about 4 months after the event and you can lose up to 20% of your hair. The good news is that it's not permanent. One thing that might stop it is to use Burdock Root tea as a hair rinse. Supplements such as Thymus gland, two 500mg; Biotin, two 5000 mcg; MSM, two 1500mg, and L-Cysteine, two 500mg daily might help.

I'm having very strange feelings…

It could be a flashback caused by toxins being released by the melting fat in your body. In fact, I've read, and experienced personally, that when the body puts on a pound of fat (for example) it takes a "snapshot" of the chemicals and hormones present in the body at that time. Emotions leave chemical tags in the body. Therefore, upon the body releasing fat stores, it "re-experiences" the feelings you had when that pound of fat was put on. Because of this, I had 3 days of really "irritable" fat to push through. Just think of it as an emotional cleansing as well as a physical one, and try to deal with the emotions that come up and try to remember when that pound of fat went on. It's a reverse type of therapy. The body is cleansing itself of not just the fat. If, at the time, some of the weight I gained was due to emotional issues/stress, now finally I would be releasing those negative things along with my fat! How great is that? The fat (a negative) is converted into energy for us to use (a positive) and the rest is let go of, released, a flushing of fat and baggage. This way when we arrive at our new body, we will be ready to really have a brand new life.

Should I be concerned about lightheadedness, weakness, tiredness?

My first 3 days on VLCD I was really tired and took a nap every day when I came home from work. Now I'm fine. The quickest way to get over this is to take a couple of 99 mg tablets of Potassium. Wal-Mart has it in the vitamin section. You will only need to take it for a short time. Your potassium level can plummet right at first because of all the water your body is releasing. It's very common to feel a little fuzzy and maybe light-headed or dizzy early on. Many have felt the same and this is the fastest fix. If your potassium is too low, it can also cause headache, tiredness, muscle weakness, and mental confusion. Too much potassium can also cause your heart to stop. But, in a healthy body, your kidneys should regulate your levels and excrete any extra you might have in the urine.

If potassium doesn't work, try eating a couple of heaped teaspoons of sugar (Simeons, p. 82).

I'm having leg cramps. What can I do?

Potassium works for this problem, too.

Why don't my muscles feel as strong as they did before I started?

In Dr. S's book on page 80, he mentions that as fat leaves the muscles, you may go through a period where it feels like your muscles have to work harder because they can't shrink in length fast enough to make up for the volume of fat reduction.

Why am I having headaches, itchy skin or a rash?

These are probably toxins being released from the fat that you are releasing. They will last as long as you don't provide other pathways for them to exit your body. One way to do this is to take a cleansing bath in the evening. Add 2 cups of Epson salts or one of baking soda and one of the Epson salts to a tub with water as hot as you can stand it and get in for 20 minutes. Make sure it comes up to your belly button or higher. AlkaSelzer Gold taken orally can help as well. Another way is through coffee enemas or colonics with a certified colon hydrotherapist. Go to **www.i-act.org** and find one in your area. Make sure that they use the LIBBE system. There are several websites with recipes for coffee enemas that can be located with a search engine if you opt for that solution. An ionic foot bath is another cleanse that can be done during the diet, but most of the electrolyte replacement drinks have ingredients that we cannot have during Phase 2, so it isn't optimal to do the foot baths without replacing the minerals that they deplete. The very best way to cleanse from toxins being released during fat reduction is a product called Natural Cellular Defense (NCD) liquid Zeolite. You can obtain it from this link: **http://tinyurl.com/Waiora**.

Is it normal to feel cold while releasing weight?

Many do report feeling unusually cold. I am one of those. Just bundle up and ride it out. It's worth it.

Step 35 – If continuing Phase 2 past 23 days, skip hCG one day a week.

If continuing Phase 2 past 23 days, skip hCG one day a week, **but continue 500 calories on that day.** This is NOT a "free" day just because you don't take a dose that day. hCG stays in your system for 3 days, according to Dr S, and eating even normally while it is in your system will cause a gain. The half-life is 33 hours. Peak concentrations of chorionic gonadotropin occur approximately 6 hours after intramuscular injection, and 16 to 20 hours after subcutaneous injection in males. One study reported that in females, it occurs after approximately 20 hours.

Do I have to skip a dose one day a week to prevent immunity?

Not if you are only doing a 23-day course of hCG. Skipping an injection 1 day per week is recommended on the 43-day protocol in order to lessen the potential for immunity, and the skipped day should always remain on the same day of the week. "Patients who require more than the minimum of 23 injections and who therefore skip one day a week in order to postpone immunity to HCG cannot have their third injections on the day before the interval. Thus if it is decided to skip Sundays, the treatment can be started on any day of the week except Thursdays. Supposing they start on Thursday, they will have their third injection on Saturday, which is also the day on which they start their 500 Calorie diet. They would then have no injection on the second day of dieting; this exposes them to an unnecessary hardship, as without the injection they will feel particularly hungry." (Simeons, p. 59)

What is the immunity that Simeons talks about?

On page 53, Dr S tells us: "The reason for limiting a course to 40 injections is that by then some patients may begin to show signs of HCG immunity. Though this phenomenon is well known, we cannot as yet define the underlying mechanism. Maybe after a certain length of time the body learns to break down and eliminate HCG very rapidly, or possibly prolonged treatment leads to some sort of counter-regulation which annuls the diencephalic effect."

How do I know if I have developed immunity?

You will know if you reach immunity because you will become ravenously hungry. What I am told is that it is the experience of wanting to eat your pillow during the night because you are SO hungry.

Anything less than that, it would not be immunity. Dr S says on page 94: "When abnormal fat is no longer being put into circulation either because it has been consumed or because immunity has set in, this is always felt by the patient as sudden, intolerable and constant hunger."

What do I do if I do develop immunity at some point?

I think that someone who hits immunity could go to 800-1000 calories a day (of VLCD foods only) for those three days after hCG is stopped. My reasoning is based on this passage in P&I:
"As soon as such patients have lost all their abnormal superfluous fat, they at once begin to feel ravenously hungry in spite of continued injections. This is because HCG only puts abnormal fat into circulation and cannot, in the doses used, liberate normal fat deposits; indeed, it seems to prevent their consumption. As soon as their statistically normal weight is reached, these patients are put on 800-1000 Calories for the rest of the treatment. The diet is arranged in such a way that the weight remains perfectly stationary and is thus continued for three days after the 23rd injection. Only then are the patients free to eat anything they please except sugar and starches for the next three weeks."

Although Dr S is referring to someone who has reached their statistically normal weight, I think that it is the same circumstance as someone who has reached immunity, since abnormal fat is no longer being released into the bloodstream. The ravenous hunger also sounds the same as immunity, and in this passage, he alludes to them as being the same circumstance:

"When a patient has consumed all his abnormal fat or, when after a full course, the injection has temporarily lost its efficacy owing to the body having gradually evolved a counter regulation, the patient at once begins to feel much more hungry and even weak. In spite of repeated warnings, some over-enthusiastic patients do not report this. However, in about two days the fact that they are being undernourished becomes visible in their faces, and treatment is then stopped at once. In such cases - and only in such cases - we allow a very slight increase in the diet, such as an extra apple, 150 grams of meat or two or three extra breadsticks during the three days of dieting after the last injection."

In that passage, he does not say 800-1000 calories, but rather some extra food that might amount to that much.

Is immunity forever if it happens to you?

Dr. S states on page 53, "After 40 daily injections it takes about six weeks before this so called immunity is lost and HCG again becomes fully effective." So, no, it is NOT forever. On pages 54-55, he goes on to instruct that the time between courses or rounds, as we sometimes call them, increases with each new round. "A second course can be started after an interval of not less than six weeks, though the pause can be more than six weeks. When a third, fourth or even fifth course is necessary, the interval between courses should be made progressively longer. Between a second and third course eight weeks should elapse, between a third and fourth course twelve weeks, between a fourth and fifth course twenty weeks and between a fifth and sixth course six months. In this way it is possible to bring about a weight reduction of 100 lbs. and more if required without the least hardship to the patient."

Step 36 – *If you remain at the same weight for four days, you may do an apple day.*

If you remain at the same weight for four days, you may do an apple day, as described on page 68-69 of "Pounds and Inches" under the second type of plateau. The instructions for an apple day are given in the next section.

Four Types of Stalls in Weight Reduction

Most hCG dieters lose more the first week, but then level out to a pound OR LESS a day thereafter. Five pounds for a week is great after the first week.

1. On page 67, Dr S explains how we lose the weight, which also could explain a stall in reduction: "The weight registered by the scale is determined by two processes not necessarily synchronized. Under the influence of HCG, fat is being extracted from the cells, in which it is stored in the fatty tissue. When these cells are empty and therefore serve no purpose, the body breaks down the cellular structure and absorbs it, but breaking up of useless cells, connective tissue, blood vessels, etc., may lag behind the process of fat-extraction. When this happens the body appears to replace some of the extracted fat with water which is retained for this purpose. As water is heavier than fat the scales may show no loss of weight, although sufficient fat has actually been consumed to make up for the deficit in the 500-Calorie diet. When then such tissue is finally broken down, the water is liberated and there is a sudden flood of urine and a marked loss of weight. This simple interpretation of what is really an extremely complex mechanism is the one we give those patients who want to know why it is that on certain days they do not lose, though they have committed no dietary error."

2. Dr. S. says that you can do an apple day if you suspect water retention and need a psychological boost. From Pounds and Inches, pages 68-69: "The second type of interruption we call a "plateau". A plateau lasts 4-6 days and frequently occurs during the second half of a full course, particularly in patients that have been doing well and whose overall average of nearly a pound per effective injection has been maintained. Those who are losing more than the average all have a plateau sooner or later. A plateau always corrects, itself, but many patients who have become accustomed to a regular daily loss get unnecessarily worried and begin to fret. No amount of explanation convinces them that a plateau does not mean that they are no longer responding normally to treatment.

In such cases we consider it permissible, for purely psychological reasons, to break up the plateau. This can be done in two ways. One is a so-called "apple day". An apple-day begins at lunch and continues until just before lunch of the following day. The patients are given six large apples and are told to eat one whenever they feel the desire though six apples is the maximum allowed. During an apple-day no other food or liquids except plain water are allowed and of water they may only drink just enough to quench an uncomfortable thirst if eating an apple still leaves them thirsty. Most patients feel no need for water and are quite happy with their six apples. Needless to say, an apple-day may never be given on the day on which there is no injection. The apple-day produces a gratifying loss of weight on the following day, chiefly due to the elimination of water. This water is not regained when the patients resume their normal 500-Calorie diet at lunch, and on the following days they continue to lose weight satisfactorily. The other way to break up a plateau is by giving a non-mercurial diuretic for one day. We use 1 tablet of hygroton.

This is simpler for the patient, but we prefer the apple-day, as we sometimes find that though the diuretic is very effective, on the following day it may take two to three days before the normal daily reduction is resumed, throwing the patient into a new fit of despair. It is useless to give either an apple-day or a diuretic unless the weight has been stationary for at least four days without any dietary error having been committed."

3. Another type of stall is identified by Dr S on page 69: "The third type of interruption in the regular loss of weight may last much longer - ten days to two weeks. Fortunately, it is rare and only occurs in very advanced cases, and then hardly ever during the first course of treatment. It is seen only in those patients who during some period of their lives have maintained a certain fixed degree of obesity for ten

years or more and have then at some time rapidly increased beyond that weight. When then in the course of treatment the former level is reached, it may take two weeks of no loss, in spite of HCG and diet, before further reduction is normally resumed."

4. The last type of stall he discusses on page 70 and it applies only to women: "The fourth type of interruption is the one which often occurs a few days before and during the menstrual period and in some women at the time of ovulation."

If you are not reducing or (heaven forbid) gaining, but don't believe that you are cheating…

It's interesting that strange things can stall you or even make you gain.

From Dr. S:
Page 67:
"Patients who have previously regularly used diuretics as a method of reducing, lose fat during the first two or three weeks of treatment which shows in their measurements, but the scale may show little or no loss because they are replacing the normal water content of their body which has been dehydrated. Diuretics should never be used for reducing."
Page 77:
"Apart from diet and cosmetics there can be a few other reasons for a small rise in weight. Some patients unwittingly take chewing gum, throat pastilles, vitamin pills, cough syrups etc., without realizing that the sugar or fats they contain may interfere with a regular loss of weight. Sex hormones or cortisone in its various modern forms must be avoided…"

Sleep

Dr S states on page 78: "Occasionally we allow a sleeping tablet or a tranquilizer, but patients should be told that while under treatment they need and may get less sleep. For instance, here in Italy where it is customary to sleep during the siesta which lasts from one to four in the afternoon most patients find that though they lie down they are unable to sleep."

However, beware of real sleep deprivation. Losing too much sleep means that your hormones are not released as they would be normally. Weight reduction seems to occur in the last 3 hours of sleep IF you get your 6 to 8 hours. I have found that the amount of sleep I get affects my weight reduction the next morning. If I get 8 or more hours, I am on track; anything less and I can stall. So be sure to get enough sleep! Several clinical studies now link sleep deprivation with weight gain:
http://tinyurl.com/sleepdeprived http://tinyurl.com/sleepdeprived2

Troubleshooting questions:

1. Did you use any nutritive oils or lotions on your skin?
2. Did you get any nutritive fats on your skin while preparing meals for others?
3. Did you eat chicken that is not breast meat or ground meat with added fillers or fat?
4. Did you eat any kind of turkey, any kind of smoked meat/fish, wrong types of fish?
5. Did you eat any meals out that might have had some unknown/hidden fat or sugar?
6. Are you cooking with Pam? Stop. It stalled one of the folks in my support group.
7. Are you using powdered Stevia that has maltodextrin or lactose in it? Change to liquid Stevia.
8. Are you using Equal (aspartame), Splenda (sucralose), or powdered Stevia packets that have maltodextrin or dextrose in it? Change to liquid Stevia.
9. Are you getting at least 8 hours of sleep per night, preferably continuous?

10. Did you take any pills that could have additives in them as fillers, or have a sugar coating?
11. Are you weighing your raw protein CAREFULLY for each/every meal?
12. Are you measuring your water to ensure intake of two liters or 64 ounces daily?
13. Are you only eating foods on Dr. Simeons' list? Sometimes, it helps to write out exactly what you ate and drank, to identify the problem.
14. Is it close to your menses or ovulation?
15. Are you at a weight that you maintained for an extended time in the past?

More suggestions to break a stall:

1. Drink MORE teas.
2. Try eating apples and ½ grapefruit instead of strawberries and oranges, which some stall on.
3. Try to walk at least a little more.
4. Try fresh spinach as your vegetable.
5. Cut out cabbage, which stalls some of us.
6. Eat nothing but organic.
7. Check your spice labels for hidden sugar or oil.
8. Drop the IM injection dosage to 125 IU. If that doesn't work, try increasing it in increments, but no more than 200 IU, unless injecting subcutaneous, and then the limit is 250 IU. Sublingual dosage should not exceed 333 IU per day, divided into 2 doses approximately 12 hours apart.
9. Start drinking an ACV cocktail 1-2 times per day.
10. Cut back on tomato or shrimp consumption if you are eating them every day.
11. Try omitting the allowed Wasa/grissini/melba toast each day.
12. Try eating meals earlier in the day.
13. Eat at least one meal each day with a large green salad.
14. If you are drinking a gallon or more of water, drink less water, but at least 64 oz daily.
15. The detox baths suggested previously can help to break a stall sometimes.
16. Here is a controversial suggestion: Try some real cream in your coffee, a piece of sugar-free dark chocolate, a bit of coconut oil, or some other small form of fat just before bed when you are on a stall. NOTE: Don't try this two days in a row, but it can work to get your weight reduction going again when used on just one day.

Hang in there. I promise that you will start reducing again. Again, I learned everything that I needed to know about stalls in nursery school. "You get what you get and you don't get upset." I once stalled for 14 full days at a former long-term weight, just as Dr S says, and it ENDED just like he said it would. Yours will, too.

Step 37 – Begin your preparation mentally for Phase 3.

I am hungry during the last few days of hCG. What could be wrong?
If you find that you are still hungry when eating the recommended amount of calories and foods for the protocol, and if you are really ravenous, you could be experiencing immunity.

I am afraid of going into P3. My greatest fear is that I will gain it all back as I have before on other diets.
You said, "My greatest fear is that I will gain it all back as I have before on other diets." You MUST relax in P3 to be successful. Zen out, as they say.

Have you ever heard this scripture? "For my sighing comes before I eat, And my groanings pour out like water. For the thing I greatly feared has come upon me. And what I dreaded has happened to me. I am not at ease, nor am I quiet. I have no rest for trouble comes." Job 3: 24-26

I believe that this can refer to our fears becoming a self-fulfilling prophecy. Think of fear as an acronym:
F alse
E vidence
A ppearing
R eal

So, let's go with these scriptures also:

"For God hath not given us the spirit of fear; but of power, and of love, and of a sound mind." 2 Timothy 1:7

"Peace I leave with you; My peace I give to you; not as the world gives do I give to you. Do not let your heart be troubled, nor let it be fearful." John 14:27

I believe that this diet was a gift from God for me and for all of us, so I also believe that trusting Him/Her/AllThatIs to care for me in P3 is just as important as doing so in P2. You can also look at it as a result of the Law of Attraction, if you believe in that. You can look at it from simply a scientific point of view and say that if you are stressed, you release cortisol, which is a fat-storing and promoting substance.

Any way that works for you to see this, it is a good thing to trust that if you are faithful to this diet, it is faithful to you. Worrying only tends to attract to you what you fear and focus on. What you focus on gets bigger, so make sure that what you are focusing on is something that you want more of.

Must I take a six-week break after 40 injections or 34 pounds released?

It is a personal decision. Dr. Simeons states that you must in order to avoid developing immunity to hCG; however, he also adds that "The only exception we make is in the case of grotesquely obese patients who may be allowed to lose an additional 5-6 lbs. if this occurs before the 40 injections are up." The Releana oral protocol does not require it. Some people are testing this method. Dr. Simeons states that if you are developing immunity, you will know it, because you will have ravenous hunger, indicating that the hCG is no longer working to suppress hunger.

Another concern is that you may not want to be on the verge of protein deficiency for a longer period of time than the maximum recommended by Dr S. In addition, taking the break gives your skin more time to shrink back up, since this seems to happen in P3/P4.

Shouldn't I be worried about sagging skin after such rapid weight reduction?

One person from my support group says that there is no loose skin after a 100 pound reduction. I myself have much less cellulite, with no hanging skin, after a 50 pound release.

You don't lose structural fat with this diet, which is why the skin does not sag as much as with other types. The normal fat stays intact and the skin usually shrinks further to return to normal in P3/P4. However, if you are still concerned, dry brushing is good for preventing loose, slack skin.
http://tinyurl.com/DrySkinBrush

Phase 3

Step 38 – One week before discontinuation of hCG, begin planning Phase 3 meals.

One week before discontinuation of hCG, begin planning Phase 3 meals with no refined sugar or starch. Do NOT limit fat, salt, or anything else, only sugar and starch are omitted. Plan in particular for much more protein, as you are on the verge of protein deficiency when beginning Phase 3.

hCG Phase 3 Recipes

Cheesy Cauliflower Mash (Mashed Potato Alternative) *A Tammy Recipe
Steamed cauliflower
1 cup sharp cheddar cheese
¼ cup half and half or sour cream
Salt and black pepper to taste
Steam the cauliflower in water until soft. Puree in blender or food processor. Add the half and half and cheddar cheese. Pour cauliflower mixture into a saucepan and heat. Add salt and pepper to taste and serve. Makes multiple servings <u>Variations</u>: Instead of cheddar, add grilled onions and blue cheese. Or mix in parmesan cheese and Italian herbs. Use less liquid and squeeze out into mounds on a cookie sheet and bake until brown. Layer with other vegetables, mushrooms, and Swiss cheese and bake like a pie.

Tzatziki Sauce
Plain Yogurt, drained
Cucumber
4 cloves Garlic
Sea Salt
Freshly Ground Black Pepper
Shred a cucumber, put it in a paper towel, and press out the water. Mix everything and you have the best Tzatziki. Refrigerate for at least 1 hour to let the tastes meld. If you really want to make true Tzatziki, buy Greek yogurt. A good brand is Total brand yogurt. There is no comparison between full fat Greek yogurt and drained American yogurt. Greek yogurt is made from Goats' milk unlike American yogurt and it makes a difference. Phase 3 variation: Add a few tablespoons of Extra Virgin Olive Oil and some fresh or dry dill to taste.

Mayonnaise
2 large Egg Yolks
3 T Lemon Juice
¼ t Sea Salt
Pinch of White Pepper
1 C Extra Light Olive Oil
Put the yolks, lemon juice, salt, and pepper into a mixing bowl and whisk until smooth and light. Then whisk the oil, a few drops at a time, into the mixture. Ensure the mixture is smooth and well integrated before pouring the next few drops of oil. The whisking will suspend the oil into the yolk mixture and

adding the oil a little at a time will keep the mixture in a state of emulsion. After about 1/3 C of the oil has been whisked in, you can speed up the pouring a bit. Ensure the mixture is back in emulsion before pouring any more oil. After all the oil has been whisked in, you have mayonnaise. This is a good time to add any extras, such as a spoonful of Dijon mustard and extra salt and black pepper if you like. Because homemade mayonnaise is mostly egg yolk, the mayonnaise will have a healthy yellow color. Store bought or machine made mayonnaise usually also contains egg whites which will lighten the color up as well as lighten up the flavor. Any you don't use immediately, put in a tightly sealed jar and refrigerate. It should stay fresh for a week.

Ranch Dressing
¾ C Mayonnaise
¼ C Buttermilk
½ t Garlic Powder
¼ t Cayenne Pepper
¼ t Fresh Cracked Black Pepper
1 Dash of Dried Minced Garlic

Phase 3 Chocolate/Chocolate Sauce *A Tammy Recipe
2 tablespoons virgin coconut oil or butter
3 tablespoons cocoa powder
Stevia to taste
Melt coconut oil or butter. Mix in cocoa powder and stevia to taste. Adjust the level of cocoa or oil to achieve desired consistency. Enjoy warm as a chocolate dipping sauce for fresh fruits.
Variations: Dip fresh fruit into chocolate sauce and refrigerate for chocolate covered raspberries, strawberries, peaches etc. Make your own homemade chocolate bark by adding chopped almonds or other nuts and refrigerate to harden. Add flavored extracts like mint, orange, almond or other flavorings to the chocolate mixture.

Zucchini Lasagna *A Tammy Recipe
Zucchini thin sliced lengthwise
12 ounce container ricotta cheese
1 8 ounce ball of mozzarella cheese
Spaghetti sauce (sugar free)
Sausage
Chopped mushrooms
1 teaspoon dried basil
Pinch of dried oregano
Parmesan cheese to taste
Salt and pepper to taste
Mix ricotta cheese with dried herbs, parmesan, salt and freshly ground black pepper. Grate the mozzarella and set aside. Layer the zucchini on the bottom of a baking dish. Smooth a layer of the ricotta mixture over the zucchini. Sprinkle with mushrooms and/or sausage, spaghetti sauce, and sprinkle with mozzarella. Repeat this procedure until you have filled the baking dish. Top with spaghetti sauce and additional mozzarella cheese. Bake lasagna in a 375 degree oven for about 30 minutes or until mozzarella is brown and bubbly on top. Makes multiple servings

Phase 3 Crustless Key Lime Pie
Yogurt
Stevia
Vegetable Glycerin

Vanilla
1 Lime, Juiced
It tastes better than key lime pie.

Cheesecake
4 Packs of Cream Cheese
Small Amount of Sour Cream
4 Eggs
1 T Vanilla
¼ To ½ C pure powdered Stevia (no fillers)
Blend cream cheese and stevia and eggs. Add vanilla. Bake in a springform pan in a water bath at 350 degrees for 1 hour. Check with a toothpick in the middle to see if is done. Cool and remove from pan. Phase 4 Variation: add peanut butter, pumpkin, maple syrup, eggnog, chocolate chips, or pureed banana to the batter.

Steak, Fish, and Chicken Marinade
Coconut Oil
Coconut Milk
Garlic

Salad Dressing
Extra Virgin Olive Oil
Virgin Coconut Oil
Garlic
Oregano
Basil
Stevia
Melt coconut oil and add fresh garlic, oregano, basil and whatever other seasonings you like.
10 minutes

Crab Salad
For the crab meat in this recipe only buy the real stuff, the kind you have to get in the refrigerated section near the meat market. DO NOT use that fake crab meat; it's full of sugar.
Equal parts of cooked lump crab meat and fresh shrimp (cooked), about ½ C each.
2 medium Tomatoes, seeded and diced
4 T fresh Cilantro, chopped fine
¼ to ½ medium yellow Onion 1015)
½ Avocado, diced
1 T Mayo, using recipe given above
Juice of ½ of a fresh Lime
Place ingredients in a bowl, mix, and salt to taste. If you like it spicy, add a sprinkle of red pepper flakes.
10 minutes

Miracle Noodles

Miracle Noodles are a product that you can use on P3 if you are missing pasta. Some have even been able to use them on P2, but that is a bit risky. My friend Tammy has written a wonderful new cookbook just for these noodles. It will be on the market very soon, so keep checking this link to purchase it: **http://tinyurl.com/MiraNoocookbook**. The noodles are available at: **http://tinyurl.com/MiraNoo**.

Even though the label may state that they are made of Yam Flour, actually they are made from a Japanese plant called konnyaku imu. In Japan, this plant is also known as an Elephant yam, so the package states yam flour noodles. However, it is different from our yams in the US. This yam is all soluble fiber and is also known as glucomannan or konjac.

Since the raw plant is 30% starch, perhaps all of it is removed in the glucomannan extraction process, to make the glucomannan more pure, as outlined in these three links:
http://tinyurl.com/Glucomannan
http://tinyurl.com/Glucomannan2
http://tinyurl.com/Glucomannan3

Step 39 – Review the Phase 3 lists of sugars and starches.

Review this Phase 3 section of the book, particularly the lists of sugars and starches. Before you start P3, READ THIS PASSAGE and heed Dr Simeons' warning. It is SO IMPORTANT to eat enough protein and calories when beginning P3. Don't be afraid to eat in P3. In fact, on page 95, Dr. Simeons warns us to:

"Beware of Over-enthusiasm

The other trouble which is frequently encountered immediately after treatment is again due to over-enthusiasm. Some patients cannot believe that they can eat fairly normally without regaining weight. They disregard the advice to eat anything they please except sugar and starch and want to play safe. They try more or less to continue the 500-Calorie diet on which they felt so well during treatment and make only minor variations, such as replacing the meat with an egg, cheese, or a glass of milk. To their horror they find that in spite of this bravura, their weight goes up. So, following instructions, they skip one meager lunch and at night eat only a little salad and drink a pot of unsweetened tea, becoming increasingly hungry and weak. The next morning they find that they have increased yet another pound. They feel terrible, and even the dreaded swelling of their ankles is back. Normally we check our patients one week after they have been eating freely, but these cases return in a few days. Either their eyes are filled with tears or they angrily imply that when we told them to eat normally we were just fooling them."

On pages 95-96, Simeons also warns of eating too little protein on P3:

"Protein deficiency

Here too, the explanation is quite simple. During treatment the patient has been only just above the verge of protein deficiency and has had the advantage of protein being fed back into his system from the breakdown of fatty tissue. Once the treatment is over there is no more HCG in the body and this process no longer takes place. Unless an adequate amount of protein is eaten as soon as the treatment is over, protein deficiency is bound to develop, and this inevitably causes the marked retention of water known as hunger- edema.

The treatment is very simple. The patient is told to eat two eggs for breakfast and a huge steak for lunch and dinner followed by a large helping of cheese and to phone through the weight the next morning. When these instructions are followed a stunned voice is heard to report that two lbs. have vanished overnight, that the ankles are normal but that sleep was disturbed, owing to an extraordinary need to pass large quantities of water. The patient having learned this lesson usually has no further trouble."

Food items that you CAN NOT have in Phase 3 include:

- potatoes
- rice
- pasta
- corn
- tortillas
- sugar (including honey, sugar, brown sugar, molasses, or any artificial sweeteners)
- breads of any kind, not even the grissini you were allowed in Phase 2
- sweet potatoes or yams
- sweeter fruits, although they seem okay for some in my support group
- chips, pretzels, crackers, or anything similar

Food items that you CAN HAVE:

- eggs
- meat of any kind prepared grilled, fried in oil, baked, as long as it isn't breaded
- cheese
- milk (preferably whole)
- cream
- any vegetable with the exception of starchy ones (see list under Starches in P3)
- some fruit (try to stay away from the really sweet ones like pineapple and grapes)
- stevia is still the sweetener of choice
- keep doing your teas, water, and so on

Normally, a whole food would not have much sugar and it is naturally-occurring in a whole food, not added refined sugar. Interestingly enough, some folks can't eat much fruit in P3 because of the sugar, even naturally-occurring, while others can eat bananas, which are not only very sweet fruit, which Simeons warns us to be careful with, but also depending on ripeness, may have some starch. As the fruit ripens, the starch turns to sugar. We all seem to be different. Not only that, but each round of hCG seems to be a bit different from the last. Do the right thing by keeping good records and learning what works for you in P3. That said, the first few days of P3, people seem more likely to have the violent fluctuations in weight that Dr S referred to, that frequently do not happen with the same food in the last week of P3.

Healthy Oils in Phase 3

Actually, the generally accepted theory that saturated fat damages your arteries and is not heart-healthy is not necessarily true, despite the 25 years of propaganda otherwise, so be sure to eat your protein-rich foods without regard to the fat in them in Phase 3. See "What if it's all been a big fat lie?" in the NY Times: **http://tinyurl.com/bigfatlie.** Or this explanation that there is no proof that saturated fat is bad: **http://tinyurl.com/notproven** While I'm on the subject, if your doctor wants to lower your cholesterol level with a statin drug, if it were me, I wouldn't. As statins prevent the liver from producing cholesterol, they also prevent it from producing a potent anti-oxidant, Co-Q-10, that is good for cardiovascular health. **http://tinyurl.com/Cholmyth** Also, studies have concluded that lipid-lowering drugs increase incidence of cancer in rodents. Here's an example: **http://tinyurl.com/StatinCancer** And there really isn't proof that high cholesterol should be treated, anyway, in my opinion. **http://tinyurl.com/cholester** Half of the people that get heart disease each year have cholesterol levels within "normal" ranges. In my opinion, C-Reactive Protein is a better marker for heart disease, since it will indicate whether or not you have inflammation.

To get healthy oils in P3, you can add coconut oil.

Isn't coconut oil one of the worst saturated fats?

You are thinking of the old style hydrogenated coconut oil. Virgin coconut oil is very healthy for you. Coconut oil has some truly unique qualities. It contains medium chain triglycerides (fatty acids), which are easier to digest because they are handled by the liver directly and can be used directly by the body as an energy source. In addition, it may benefit weight management because it can rev up your thyroid to stimulate the metabolism and give you energy. Some even use a bit of it in P2, but it's a risky thing to try unless you are stalled. Coconut oil is excellent for cooking and baking, and is also used externally as a skin moisturizer and hair conditioner. Lots of research and peer-reviewed articles here: **http://www.coconutoil.com/**

Alternatively, you can get pure MCT oil, which will have the same effects. Whatever you do, don't try to skimp on calories or eat low-fat/non-fat products or you WILL gain. Eat to satisfaction. If you do gain some, have eggs for breakfast, lots of cheese and protein on a big salad with oily dressing for lunch and a huge steak for dinner with berries and heavy cream for dessert. I swear it works.

Sugar in Phase 3

Sugar-free on a product label means that it has no sucrose. It may, however, have fructose, molasses, honey, corn syrup, or sugar alcohols, as well as artificial sweeteners such as sucralose, aspartame, or saccharin. All you can really be sure of is that it has no sucrose. To wean yourself off of sugar, you may find it helpful to take a gram or two a day of omega 3 fish oils, to reduce the cravings. Placing 500 mg of L-Glutamine from an opened capsule under the tongue to absorb sublingually also will help. If it is Candida driving the sweet or starch cravings, you will need to treat that underlying cause with either Candida-G (Phase 2) or FermPlus (Phase 3) to get rid of them.

The USDA web site says that the United States is the largest consumer of sweeteners, including high fructose corn syrup. There is no doubt that we have a major problem with sugar consumption in this country.

Does anyone know which fruits are supposed to be the "sweet fruits" to which Dr. Simeons refers?

Based on a chart that breaks out fruits by glycemic impact, sweet fruits are considered to be any and all dried or dehydrated fruits because they become concentrated when all the liquid is removed as well as raw, fresh pomegranates, passion fruits, black currants, sweet cherries, bananas, dates, figs, mangoes, jackfruits, breadfruits, crabapples, cherimoyas, persimmons, prunes, raisins, and grapes.

Fruit Sugar Content and Glycemic Load

To find the sugar content or glycemic load of any food, use: **http://www.Nutritiondata.com** or **http://www.foodfacts.com**.

Type Of Fresh Raw Fruit	Sugar Content as % of Weight	Glycemic Load	Okay for P3?
Date, deglet noor	63.4	39	NO
Date, medjool	66.5	39	NO
Persimmon, native	Unk	15	No
Jackfruit	Unk	10	No
Breadfruit	11.0	9	No
Banana (also starch)	12.2	8	No
Crabapple	Unk	7	No
Black Currant	Unk	6	No
Cherimoya	Unk	6	No
Passion Fruit	11.2	6	No
Pomegranate	13.7	6	No
Grape, seedless	15.5	6	No
Grape, sweet	16.2	6	No
Fig	16.3	6	No
Persimmon, Japanese	12.5	5	No
Sweet Cherry	12.8	5	No
Mango (also starch)	14.8	5	No
Elderberry	Unk	4	Maybe
Orange, Valencia	Unk	4	Maybe
Red Currant	7.4	4	Maybe
Mulberry	8.1	4	Maybe

Type Of Fresh Raw Fruit	Sugar Content as % of Weight	Glycemic Load	Okay for P3?
Orange, navel	8.5	4	Maybe
Sour Cherry	8.5	4	Maybe
Guava (also starch)	8.9	4	Maybe
Kiwi (bit of starch)	9.0	4	Maybe
Apricot	9.2	4	Maybe
Clementine	9.2	4	Maybe
Kumquat	9.4	4	Maybe
Blueberry	10.0	4	Maybe
Pineapple, extra sweet	10.3	4	Maybe
Mandarin Orange	10.6	4	Maybe
Tangerine	10.6	4	Maybe
Loquat	Unk	3	Yes
Blackberry	4.9	3	Yes
Grapefruit, pink and red	6.9	3	Yes
Cantaloupe	7.9	3	Yes
Peach	8.4	3	Yes
Orange	9.4	3	Yes
Pear	9.8	3	Yes
Pineapple	9.8	3	Yes
Plum	9.9	3	Yes
Apple	10.4	3	Yes
Avocado	0.7	2	Yes
Lime	1.7	2	Yes
Lemon	2.5	2	Yes
Cranberry	4.0	2	Yes
Starfruit	4.0	2	Yes
Raspberry	4.4	2	Yes
Strawberry	4.9	2	Yes
Casaba Melon	5.7	2	Yes
Gooseberry	5.9	2	Yes
Papaya	5.9	2	Yes
Prickly Pear	6.0	2	Yes
Watermelon	6.2	2	Yes
Pear, Asian	7.0	2	Yes
Grapefruit, white	7.3	2	Yes
Honeydew Melon	8.1	2	Yes
Oheloberry	Unk	1	Yes
Olives, black, ripe	0.0	1	Yes
Olives, green	0.5	1	Yes
Tomato	2.6	1	Yes

101 Names for Sugar

Typically, when ingredients are listed on a product, they must be listed from largest amount down to smallest amount found in that product. Do not be fooled into thinking there is very little sugar in an item if it is not listed near the beginning. Often you will find three or four of the following aliases in the ingredient listing, meaning that the product may be mostly sugar!

Added sugars in processed foods can be found under the following names:

1. Agave Syrup
2. Amasake
3. Any name ending in "ose" or "ol" or "syrup" (except for sucralose, which is Splenda)
4. Bar Sugar
5. Barbados Sugar
6. Barley Malt
7. Blackstrap Molasses
8. Black Sugar
9. Brown Sugar
10. Cane Juice
11. Cane Juice Crystals
12. Cane Sugar
13. Caramel
14. Caramel Coloring
15. Castor Sugar
16. Confectioner's Sugar
17. Corn Sweetener
18. Corn Syrup
19. Corn Syrup Solids
20. Crystallized Cane Juice
21. D-mannose
22. Date Sugar
23. Demerara
24. Demerara Sugar
25. Dehydrated Cane Juice
26. Dehydrated Cane Juice Crystals
27. Dextran
28. Dextrin
29. Dextrine
30. Dextrose (glucose)
31. Disaccharides
32. Evaporated Cane Juice
33. Evaporated Cane Juice Sugar
34. Florida crystals (a trademarked name)
35. Free Flowing Brown Sugars
36. Fructose
37. Fruit Juice Concentrate
38. Galactose
39. Galatactose
40. Glucose
41. Glucose Syrup
42. Golden Syrup
43. Granulated Sugar
44. Grape Sugar
45. Grape Sweetener
46. High Fructose Corn Syrup (HFCS)

47. Honey
48. Hydrolysed Starch
49. Hydrogenated Glucose Syrup
50. Hydrogenated Starch Hydrolysates (HSH)
51. Invert Sugar
52. Isomalt
53. Levulose
54. Lactitol
55. Lactose
56. Malt
57. Malt Extract
58. Malt Syrup
59. Maltodextrin
60. Maltitol
61. Maltose
62. Maple Syrup
63. Molasses
64. Monosaccharide
65. Muscovado
66. Organic Dehydrated Cane Juice
67. Panocha
68. Polysaccharide
69. Powdered Sugar
70. Rapadura
71. Raw Cane Crystals
72. Raw Honey
73. Raw Sugar
74. Refiner's Syrup
75. Ribose
76. Rice Extract
77. Rice Malt
78. Rice Syrup
79. Saccharide
80. Saccharose
81. Sorghum
82. Sorghum Syrup
83. Sucanat
84. Succanat
85. Sucrose
86. Sugar
87. Sweetener
88. Syrup
89. Table Sugar
90. Treacle
91. Turbinado
92. Turbinado Sugar
93. Unbleached Crystallized Evaporated Cane Juice
94. Unbleached Evaporated Sugar Cane Juice Crystals
95. Unbleached Sugar Cane
96. Unrefined Cane Juice Crystals

97.   Washed Cane Juice Crystals
98.   White Grape Juice
99.   Yellow Sugar
100.   Xylose
101.   Xyulose

Be aware that there are many food items that you would not think of as having added sugar that in fact do. I have found hardly any Worcestershire sauce, commercial broths or bouillons or even such items as fish marinade that didn't contain MSG, cornstarch, carrots, potato starch, sugar, or high fructose corn syrup in the ingredients.

I did find some brands of bacon that do not have sugar: Kroger and Gwaltany's (although not Nitrate-Free). Strangely, Gwaltany's hot dogs have more sugar than other brands I've seen. Go figure!?!

Almost all commercial brands of peanut butter have sugar added. I never thought about that until I saw sugar-free on one. Also, imitation crab (surimi) or other imitation seafood is usually made of herring, but contains added sugar or starch and other additives and therefore is not allowed on Phase 3.

Starches in Phase 3

So many people think that Phase 3 is Atkins and that all carbs are starches. This is totally untrue. I must respectfully disagree with the assertion that "Starches = Carbohydrates". While it is true that all refined sugar and starch are carbohydrates, all carbohydrates are NOT refined sugar and/or starch and some are mostly fiber. I believe that Dr S wanted patients to avoid high glycemic index foods for P3, although the term was not used back then. To be clear, the current standard (since 1997) for glycemic effect (blood glucose raising potential) takes into consideration not only the GI rating, but also the amount of the serving, to estimate the glycemic load (glycemic index times the carbohydrate content per serving size) based on both the quality and quantity of the food. If a standard serving of a food is larger, then that would raise the glycemic load, so both amount and GI rating of a food figure into whether you would eat it in P3.

Phase 3 isn't Atkins induction, although some do use it as a rough guide. If it was, it wouldn't allow fruit. Dr. S only says to avoid the sweeter ones. You don't have to avoid all carbs. You simply do not eat refined sugar or starch at all. That being said, many Atkins recipes are good for Phase 3. Many non-Atkins recipes are, too, if they omit refined sugar and starch.

For example, some carbs are fibrous (non-starchy, mostly cellulose) and some are starchy:

Fibrous Carbohydrates	Carbs in 100 Grams	Glycemic Load	Starchy Carbohydrates	Carbs in 100 Grams	Glycemic Load
Mustard Greens	2.1	0	Rutabagas	8.7	4
Sour Pickles	2.3	0	White Onions	9.6	4
Watercress	1.3	1	Beets	10.0	4
Cucumber	2.2	1	Winter Butternut Squash	10.5	4
Dill Pickles	2.6	1	Waterchestnuts	12.3	4
Nopales	3.3	1	Winter Acorn Squash	14.6	4
Lettuce	3.3	1	Shiitake Mushrooms	13.8	5
Summer Scallop Squash	3.4	1	Broadbeans	10.1	6
Radishes	3.5	1	Hominy / Grits	14.3	6
Spinach	3.7	1	English Peas	15.6	6
Summer Zucchini Squash	3.9	1	Parsnips	17.0	6
Celery	4.0	1	Lentils	19.5	6
Green Peppers	4.2	1	Navy Beans	15.0	7
Sauerkraut	4.3	1	Jerusalem Artichokes	17.4	7
Summer Crookneck or Straightneck Squash	4.3	1	Sweet Potatoes	17.7	7
Turnip Greens	4.4	1	Bulgur Wheat	18.6	7

Fibrous Carbohydrates	Carbs in 100 Grams	Glycemic Load	Starchy Carbohydrates	Carbs in 100 Grams	Glycemic Load
Vegetable Juice, Canned	4.5	1	Split Peas	20.5	7
Jalapenos	4.7	1	Lima Beans	20.9	7
Turnips	5.1	1	Red Beans	21.8	7
Arugula	3.7	2	Sweet Pickles	21.0	8
Swiss Chard	4.1	2	Black Beans	23.7	8
Asparagus	4.1	2	Potatoes	20.1	9
Cauliflower	4.2	2	Quinoa	21.3	10
Radicchio	4.5	2	Chickpeas (Garbanzo Beans)	27.4	10
Collard Greens	4.9	2	Brown Rice	23.0	11
Okra	4.9	2	Spelt	26.4	11
Cabbage	5.5	2	Yams	27.0	11
Yellow Pepper	6.3	2	Couscous	23.2	12
Winter Spaghetti Squash	6.5	2	Corn	25.9	12
Winter Hubbard Squash	6.5	2	Barley	28.2	12
Red Peppers	6.6	2	Pinto Beans	30.9	12
Yellow Onions	7.9	2	Taro	34.6	14
Pumpkin	8.1	2	White Rice	28.2	15
Eggplant	8.1	2	Spaghetti	30.6	16
Carrots	8.2	2	Whole Wheat English Muffins	40.4	18
Mushrooms (except Shiitake)	5.3	3	Whole Wheat Bread	41.3	19
Kale	5.6	3	Yucca (Cassava)	38.1	20
Kohlrabi	6.7	3	Whole Wheat Rolls	51.1	26
Snowpeas	6.8	3	Whole Wheat Pita	55.0	27
Brussels Sprouts	7.1	3	Whole Wheat Crackers	68.6	35
Broccoli	7.2	3	Whole Buckwheat Groat Flour	70.6	37
Green Onions	7.3	3	Oatmeal	69.0	39
Green Beans	7.9	3	Millet	72.9	44
Jicama	8.2	3	Arrowroot Flour	88.1	59
Globe Artichoke	12.0	3	Shredded Wheat, non-sweetened / sweetened	79.9 / 81.2	45 / 51

I think that the difference between starchy carbs and non-starchy carbs should be obvious from the chart above. If you stick with vegetables and grains with Glycemic Load under 4, you will have no problems, as long as you stay with a 3.5 ounce portion (100 grams). The portion size can change the

Glycemic Load. For instance, if you eat 100 grams of hubbard squash, the Glycemic Load is 2, but if you eat 236 grams, it is 5.

Carbs are pretty much the total of the sugars, fiber, and starch in a food. Therefore, you can look at the carb count on a label, subtract the fiber count and the sugar count, and the remainder is the starch count. Take a look at the potato nutrition label on this page: **http://tinyurl.com/PotatoStarch**

You can see from the Nutrition Facts box that there are 63 grams of total carbs, 7 of which are fiber and 4 of which are sugar. If you subtract the total fiber and sugar (11 grams), you will get 52 grams, which just so happens to almost exactly match the 51.6 grams of starch listed in the larger section below called Nutrition Information, in the Carbohydrates subsection. So this is an easy way to estimate the starch in any product with a label. If you are dealing with a whole food, then the process that we just used with looking up the nutritional data for the potato will work.

Another way that you can see if what you want to eat contains starch it to use the iodine test. Take a little bit of the food that you want to test and put a drop of iodine on it. If it turns very dark, it has starch. However, don't eat the part of the food that has iodine on it from the testing.

Even foods we think of as healthy may have starch. Chickpeas (which is what hummus is made from) appear to be almost half starch, while wheat is two-thirds starch as a comparison. Dietary fiber and starch concentrations for extruded chickpeas were 8.3 and 46.3 g/100 g DM, respectively, and for extruded wheat were 10.1 and 66.9 g/100 g DM, respectively.

The starchy foods you need to avoid completely are:
Bread, crackers, rolls, cookies, pizza, breakfast cereals, pancakes, waffles, rice, pasta, potatoes, snack food, fat-free or sugar free frozen yogurt, corn, potatoes, or peas.

Vegetables that are considered dense starches are:
Acorn squash, artichokes (Jerusalem), banana squash beets, beans (other than green beans), butternut squash, corn, legumes, parsnips, peas, potatoes, sweet potatoes, and yams.

Carbohydrates that contain little or NO starch:
Artichokes (globe, the green ones), asparagus, avocados, bamboo shoots, beet greens, broccoli, brussels sprouts, cabbage, capers, carrots, cauliflower, celery, collard greens, cucumbers, dandelion greens, eggplant, endive, greens, green beans, horseradish, hubbard squash, kale, kohlrabi, leeks, lettuce, mayonnaise, mustard, mustard greens, mushrooms, okra, olives, onions, parsley, pumpkin, peppers, radishes, rhubarb, rutabagas, sorrel, spaghetti squash, spinach, sprouts, string beans, swiss chard, tomatoes, turnips, turnip greens, vinegar, watercress, and wax beans.

You can use **http://www.Nutritiondata.com/** to look for starch content of foods. With regard to these starch ratings, a number of the vegetables that according to their ratings, should be safe to eat, when tested with iodine, can react showing a great deal of starch, and some don't show any at all despite these ratings stating high in starch. Garlic powder, for example, rated very high in starch; however, I've tested it with iodine and never discovered any starch. I decided that the iodine test is the best indicator of starch, for me. But of course, there is the difference in starch in plants, depending on how ripe it is when you test it – or (in the case of fruit) whether it was tree ripened or stored in an unripe state in cold storage, for months before being put on the supermarket shelves. This makes a huge difference, since the starch in the fruit never gets a chance to turn to sugar.

Starch Content of Selected Foods

Eggs, fats and oils, meat, fish, herbs and spices (unless starch has been added to a mixture), cheeses (unless pre-shredded, which sometimes have starch added to prevent sticking), milk, carbonated drinks, juices, and alcoholic beverages do not contain starch.

Flours, rices, and grains DO contain starches, EXCEPT for almond flour, which contains 1.03 grams of starch in every 100 grams, and coconut flour, which contains none. Here is the research backing the assertion that coconut flour is NOT starch: **http://tinyurl.com/coconutflour** lists coconut meat, dried, non-sweetened as 0.0 grams of starch in 100 grams. Coconut flour is made from this substance.

Fruits in general have only trace amounts of starch, if that, except for these notable exceptions: bananas, for which the starch content falls and the sugar content rises on ripening, guava, which contains a barely detectable amount, and kiwi fruit and mangoes, which have a bit more.

Vegetables that have over 5% starch include: beans other than green beans, corn, garlic, new potatoes, parsnips, plantains, potatoes, sweet potatoes, and yams.

Any beans, peas, or lentils have too much starch to be suitable for Phase 3, EXCEPT green beans, which have 2.6% starch, and runner beans, which have less than 1%. Mung bean sprouts have almost 2% starch and are probably okay. Tofu has less than 1% starch, but fresh/frozen cooked soybeans have almost 5%, which is close to the 5% limit. You can try those if you wish, but avoid if you gain.

Peas, particularly canned or processed peas, are too high in starch for Phase 3. Black-eyed peas (technically a bean), besan flour, chick pea flour, chick peas, and hummus are other items that are too high in starch.

Nuts and seeds with less than 1% starch are: Brazil nuts (0.7), coconut (0), coconut milk (0), flax seeds (0), Macadamia nuts (0.8), Pine nuts (0.1), sesame seeds (0.5), tahini paste (0.5), and walnuts (0.7). These are safe for P3. Sesame seeds do vary, however. If both dried and decorticated, they have no starch, but if not that particular type, they have too much starch for P3, around 10%. If you don't know what type that you have, it is best to discontinue both tahini paste and sesame seeds if you gain on P3.

Nuts and seeds with 5% or less starch are: almonds (2.7), hazelnuts (2), pecans (1.5), and pistachio nuts (2.5). These may be safe for some people to use in P3, but for others, might be problematic.

Nuts and seeds with more than 5% starch are: cashews (13.2), chestnuts (29.6), peanut butter (6.4) and peanuts (6), (which are technically legumes and not nuts), pumpkin seeds (pepitas) (12.9), sunflower seeds (16.3), safflower seeds (34), chia seeds (6), and watermelon seed kernels (15.3). These are very unlikely to work in P3 and almost always cause a gain, although some can tolerate small amounts of peanuts or natural peanut butter.

Ice cream alone has less than 1% starch, but you must be concerned with the added sugar unless you make your own, which you certainly can. Pudding has too much starch, over 19% for instant.

Anything that can have a filler substance or a thickening agent will usually have starch in it. For instance, luncheon or deli meats that are not cut from the original meat, sausages, regular cocoa powder, Ovaltine powder, or any kind of sauces are items that you would not think have starch, but they do, and too much for Phase 3. Bouillon cubes are a strange case. Beef flavor has only trace amounts of starch, but chicken and vegetable flavors have too much to be used on Phase 3.

Step 40 – Record your weight on your last injection or sublingual dose day.
Record your weight on your last injection or sublingual dose day.

Step 41 – Continue 500 calories for 72 hours after the last injection.
Continue 500 calories for 72 hours after the last injection or dose. You may continue to lose on these days. Sometimes, there is confusion about this because in one part of the book, he states 3 days. However, he makes it crystal clear when he says on page 98: "After 3rd injection, 500 Calorie diet to be continued until 72 hours after the last injection."

Step 42 – Review the sample Phase 3 menus.
Review the sample Phase 3 menu. Do NOT continue 500 calories after this. It is very important to eat MUCH more food and in particular, protein, for three weeks. Eat foods that were not allowed in Phase 2, but still do not have refined sugar or starch. Do NOT be afraid of fat. Use full-fat products, NOT low-fat or non-fat.

Phase 3 Sample Menu
Here is a typical day in Phase 3 for me:
Coffee with cream
3 egg Omelet with 2 slices sharp cheese sometimes with homemade salsa or a veggie like asparagus or spinach
Pink Lady Apple with 1 Tablespoon Peanut Butter sometimes, but limit this, since it is 6.4% starch
2 cups of homemade Chili with tomatoes and onions with cheese
Honeycrisp Apple
Coffee with cream
Several (maybe 3) Tacos made with sour cream and salsa with cheese, wrapped in lettuce
Okra and Tomatoes (Rotel)
Homemade Cheesecake without sugar and no crust (one or two slices, depending on hunger)
Hot tea or cold sparkling water, sometimes flavored, sometimes with Stevia

Hope that this helps anyone worried about starting P3. I have been on P4 for months and this morning, I was still below LIW.

Step 43 – Continue to weigh yourself daily in Phase 3.
Continue to weigh yourself daily in Phase 3. I used to tell folks to eat to satisfaction, but some folks could not drop the dieting mentality and ate 1500 calories or less on P3, which caused them to gain. This is the number one most frequently seen problem in P3, not eating enough, or going back to eating habits such as eating fake food or low-fat or no-fat foods, which strangely enough, causes gains, not losses or maintenance. Don't forget, your body has become accustomed to having 2500-3000 calories in the bloodstream while you were on hCG. This causes it to shut down your metabolism as if it senses a famine, if it gets substantially less than it is now accustomed to handling.

The easiest way to maintain in P3 with little to no "steak days" needed is to eat twice as many grams of fat and protein as grams of carbs, eating in your range of calories that will maintain your current weight according to the online calculator link in the next question. In other words, eat the same number of grams of protein and fat, then half that many grams of carbs. Let's say that your calorie total is 1500 calories. That would mean that you would need 100 grams of pure protein in your diet (not 100 grams of a protein source, which might only have 25 grams of pure protein), 100 grams of fat, and 50 grams of carbohydrate. This can be worked out by realizing that fat has 9 calories per gram; carbs and protein have 4 calories per gram. That means that if you have 1 gram each of fat and protein, you have 13 calories. If you have ½ gram of carbs, that is 2 calories. To maintain that ratio, you can divide the calories you need to maintain by 15 to get the number of grams of fat and protein. The carbs grams are half that much. For 1500 calories, dividing by 15 gives 100, so you'd eat 100 grams of fat, 100 grams of protein, and 50 grams of carbs, none of which should be sugary or starchy, of course, but rather fibrous vegetables and less sweet fruits for P3. 2000 calories would mean that you'd eat 133 grams of fat and the same number of protein grams, with 66.5 grams of carbs to make the 2000 calories.

How do I know how many calories I should be eating on Phases 3 or 4?

Use **http://tinyurl.com/caloriecal** to determine how many calories you should eat to maintain your LIW or LDW reached in Phase 2. The only reason that I tell you to do this is that I used to tell folks to eat to satisfaction, but some were still so out of touch with what a normal amount of food to eat really is, that they ate too little. I remind you that the number one problem that we see in my support group in P3 is that people eat too little food, and they gain from it. I know, it is counter-intuitive, but that is the truth of it. Once those same folks eat more, they maintain easily.

How do I determine my body frame size?

Wrap your thumb and fingers around your smallest part of your wrist. If your longest finger overlaps your thumb, you have a Small Frame. If your fingers barely touch, you have a Medium Frame. If your fingers don't touch, you have a Large Frame.

How can I calculate my ideal weight?

Calculate your body's frame size as described above and determine your ideal weight by using **http://tinyurl.com/bestweight**

Can I lose more weight on Phase 3?

This is not advised, because it is always at the expense of normal fat. See page 93 of Pounds and Inches referenced in the next step. Using Dr Simeons' other book "Man's Presumptuous Mind" as a reference, the section on obesity makes it clear that he does not believe that the abnormal fat deposits are touched except in the presence of hCG or the absence of normal fat to draw from, since that is the fat that is in the "current account" and "liquid" in the "money" sense for use.

Can I have alcohol on Phase 3?

Simeons allows an occasional glass of wine with a meal on Phase 3.

Step 44 – If you weigh more than 2 pounds over your last injection weight…

If you weigh more than 2 pounds over your last injection weight or last sublingual dose weight on any day, you must do a steak day on that day as described on pages 92-93 of "Pounds and Inches". Do not wait. Do it that day. If you wait, it most likely will not work to remove the extra weight.

If you absolutely cannot make it to at least 4:00 pm before eating, even with drinking lots of hot beverages, then you can try eating the apple or tomato for lunch and then the steak for dinner, which still seems to work as well as waiting for dinner for both, at least for some people. Eat a huge two pound steak if you can find one.

Dr. S states on pages 92-93:
"As long as their weight stays within two pounds of the weight reached on the day of the last injection, patients should take no notice of any increase but the moment the scale goes beyond two pounds, even if this is only a few ounces, they must on that same day entirely skip breakfast and lunch but take plenty to drink. In the evening they must eat a huge steak with only an apple or a raw tomato. Of course this rule applies only to the morning weight. Ex-obese patients should never check their weight during the day, as there may be wide fluctuations and these are merely alarming and confusing.

It is of utmost importance that the meal is skipped on the same day as the scale registers an increase of more than two pounds and that missing the meals is not postponed until the following day. If a meal is skipped on the day in which a gain is registered in the morning this brings about an immediate drop of often over a pound. But if the skipping of the meal - and skipping means literally skipping, not just having a light meal - is postponed the phenomenon does not occur and several days of strict dieting may be necessary to correct the situation.

Most patients hardly ever need to skip a meal. If they have eaten a heavy lunch they feel no desire to eat their dinner, and in this case no increase takes place. If they keep their weight at the point reached at the end of the treatment, even a heavy dinner does not bring about an increase of two pounds on the next morning and does not therefore call for any special measures. Most patients are surprised how small their appetite has become and yet how much they can eat without gaining weight. They no longer suffer from an abnormal appetite and feel satisfied with much less food than before. In fact, they are usually disappointed that they cannot manage their first normal meal, which they have been planning for weeks.

Losing more Weight

An ex-patient should never gain more than two pounds without immediately correcting this, but it is equally undesirable that more than two lbs. be lost after treatment, because a greater loss is always achieved at the expense of normal fat. Any normal fat that is lost is invariably regained as soon as more food is taken, and it often happens that this rebound overshoots the upper two lbs. limit."

I'm vegetarian. How can I do a "Steak Day"?

What do you do on a steak day if you don't eat steak? Try another high protein source.
One such person in our support group only ate fish, so she used that. Well, it worked. She ate nothing all day and had cod with tomatoes for dinner – drank lots of liquids and the next morning was below her LIW. Three days later, she was only .4 lb above her last LIW.

Step 45 – If you suspect that you have edema…

If you suspect that you have edema (water retention) caused by insufficient protein, do the eggs-steak-cheese day as described on page 96 of "Pounds and Inches":

"The patient is told to eat two eggs for breakfast and a huge steak for lunch and dinner followed by a large helping of cheese and to phone through the weight the next morning. When these instructions are followed a stunned voice is heard to report that two lbs. have vanished overnight, that the ankles are normal but that sleep was disturbed, owing to an extraordinary need to pass large quantities of water. The patient having learned this lesson usually has no further trouble."

Phase 4

Step 46 – After completing three weeks of no refined sugar or starches, you may proceed to Phase 4.

After completing three weeks of no refined sugar or starches, you may proceed to Phase 4, very gradually adding small amounts of sugars and starches. Dr. Simeons requires three weeks of Phase 4 before beginning your second round of Phase 2, if needed. He assumed that people needing more than one round would do long rounds, rather than shorter 23-dose ones, but some have done serial short rounds to avoid immunity from the longer rounds. Dr Simeons stated on page 54: "Patients who need only 23 injections may be injected daily, including Sundays, as they never develop immunity."

Therefore, although P4 is increased on each subsequent round when doing rounds of 40 doses, for 23-dose rounds, 6 weeks (3 weeks of P3, 3 weeks of P4) is sufficient between each round.

Following is a handy table of how much time to use between the longer 40-dose rounds:

Between Rounds	Phase 3 (No sugar or starch)	Phase 4
1 and 2	3 weeks	3 weeks
2 and 3	3 weeks	5 weeks
3 and 4	3 weeks	9 weeks
4 and 5	3 weeks	17 weeks
5 and 6	3 weeks	23 weeks
Any subsequent rounds	3 weeks	23 weeks

Approach Phase 4, the rest of your life, as a great adventure in finding out just what you can eat and maintain, and in finding out how your appetite and food preferences have changed. Dr Simeons states to add back starches very gradually in very small amounts, always controlled by morning weighing. I would try **one** starch or sugar at a time, in **small** amounts. If you gain the next day, cut out starch and sugar the next day to allow the gain to leave again. If that does not return you to within two pounds of LIW, then do a steak day the next day as you would in P3. I believe that steak days are a gift from Dr Simeons that can be used for life to maintain the weight as needed. Then try again and see which foods cause a gain and which do not, for you. This process, along with good records, will allow you to know which ones to which your particular body is sensitive. You can be careful not to eat those two days in a row, although things can change for the better as time goes on.

I would suggest introducing the following as your first starches and sweeter fruits that you add in P4:

Food	Amount to Start
White Potato	1/2 cup
Sweet Potato	1/2 cup
Rice	1/2 cup
Beans	1/2 cup
Corn	1/2 cup
Grapes	Small bunch
Sweet Cherries	1/2 cup
Banana	One

138

After you are maintaining easily while using these foods for a couple of weeks, you can carefully begin to introduce others, such as oatmeal, pasta, bread, or sweets with refined sugar or dried fruit. **Continue to avoid the combination of fat and starch except for an occasional indulgence.** Either of these is fine in moderation, but large amounts of both simultaneously can be risky. I have maintained in Phase 4 with no problems, for months, until I could start another round.

However, one thing that I have to watch out for is stress. I have to keep my stress levels moderate. If I allow stress to pile up, I notice that I feel very differently toward food and tend to turn to it even when I am not hungry, so stress management has been essential for me, because I don't crave foods or want unhealthy foods unless I don't manage my stress levels with EFT and activity. I enjoy bananas that have been pureed more than I enjoy ice cream now; my tastes have changed so much. Sometimes I use Tammy's Chocolate Sauce from her book on them just as I would on ice cream. Yum!

After Phase 4, you may begin another round if you are not at goal weight yet.

Do I do the loading days on subsequent courses after the first?

Yes, you do, or at least eat normally, since Dr S says that it is a fundamental mistake to start the 500 calories on the first day of hCG administration. Simeons was very specific about everything else that should be different on subsequent courses or "rounds" of hCG. In addition, he states on page 79: "If an interruption of treatment lasting more than four days is necessary, the patient must increase his diet to at least 800 Calories by adding meat, eggs, cheese, and milk to his diet after the third day, as otherwise he will find himself so hungry and weak that he is unable to go about his usual occupation. If the interval lasts less than two weeks the patient can directly resume injections and the 500-Calorie diet, *but if the interruption lasts longer he must again eat normally until he has had his third injection.*" This clearly indicates that subsequent rounds of hCG after breaks of longer than two weeks require loading again, or at the very least, interpreting what Dr. S said very literally, eating a normal amount of food instead of the VLCD for the first two days of injections.

If you have reached your goal weight, CELEBRATE!!!

How to Stay Slim Afterwards for Life

The following sections are meant for you to use during the rest of your life to help to prevent gaining weight again, both because of the overconsumption of refined carbohydrates and the additives in most of our food, including fat-free or low-fat processed foods, soy, high fructose corn syrup, and monosodium glutamate (MSG).

Fat-Free Really Means Sugar-Full

What does Fat-Free on a label mean, anyway? Surprise! What it does NOT mean is "free of fat". Fat-free or trans-fat-free means that each serving contains less than half a gram of fat or trans fat. It could be .49 gram and still be considered zero. I'll bet you have wondered why some foods seem to have impossibly small "serving" sizes. Now you know why.

This will go against everything that you've been told for years, but those fat-free products are more likely to make you gain weight again, for a couple of reasons:
- Fat induces satiety and makes you satisfied with what you have eaten. For this reason, a shortage of fat in your diet is likely to cause increased appetite.
- Another problem with these products is that when fat is removed, some form of refined carbohydrate is almost always added. If it's fat-free, you can bet it is sugar-full! As we know from Gary Taubes' research, that is exactly what needs to be avoided as much as possible to avoid obesity.

For example, on the Land 'o Lakes Fat Free Half & Half, corn syrup is the second ingredient.
Just take a look at the list of ingredients on the container:
Nonfat Milk, Corn Syrup, Cream (Adds a Trivial Amount of Fat), Artificial Color (an Ingredient Not Normally Found in Half & Half), Sodium Citrate, Dipotassium Phosphate, Mono & Diglycerides (Adds a Trivial Amount of Fat), Carrageenan, Vitamin A Palmitate.

A Word about Soy Products

While I am on controversial subjects, I'll give you my opinions, based on research, about eating a lot of soy products. Although currently perceived in the mainstream as healthy replacements for animal protein and milk, soy products have several downsides associated with them. Small amounts of Bragg's Amino Acids as seasonings probably won't have significant effects, but I see people and children drinking large quantities of soy milk every day, thinking that they are doing something good for themselves and healthy for their bodies, when in fact, they are introducing an endocrine disruptor into their bodies that could have dire consequences later on.

As an example, it saddens me, as more and more men need to buy Viagra to function sexually **http://tinyurl.com/soytruth4 http://tinyurl.com/soytruth5** and are developing breasts **http://tinyurl.com/soytruth3** and impaired sperm **http://tinyurl.com/soytruth2**, that few people realize that one of the effects of such large quantities of soy, which contains phytoestrogens, is to increase estrogen in the body. Now, eating large quantities of meats or milks with hormones in them because of the livestock having received hormonal injections is not any better, but eating protein and milk sources free of rBST/rBGH can avoid this problem altogether. A book by Kaayla T. Daniel, *The Whole Soy Story: The Dark Side of America's Favorite Health Food* explains more: **http://tinyurl.com/Soystory**

140

Soy also can have effects on thyroid function. So can broccoli or any cruciferous veggies if eaten excessively. And the most concerning of all: soy can impair fertility or ability to carry to term in mice: **http://tinyurl.com/soytruth**

High Fructose Corn Syrup Concerns

Read your labels carefully. I will NEVER buy anything with this ingredient. It is made from corn syrup using enzymes to increase the fructose. Fructose can raise triglyceride levels and increase risk of heart disease. The corn it is made from is usually GMO. **http://tinyurl.com/HFCS10**

And now, to top it all off, HCFS has been found to be contaminated with mercury:
http://tinyurl.com/HFCSmercury
http://tinyurl.com/HFCSmercury2

You may have seen a television advertisement campaign that the corn industry has recently started to counter the increasingly widespread knowledge of HFCS concerns. It's quite clever and directs you to the site: **http://www.sweetsurprise.com**. The funding sources (food producers that use HFCS) for the clinical studies that are cited on this site have been called into question:
http://tinyurl.com/HFCS11 The corn industry wants you to believe that their HFCS product has been maligned. You can read and decide if these clinical studies, not paid for by the food industry, are more credible and vote with your pocketbook:

Bantle, J., et al. (2000). Effects of dietary fructose on plasma lipids in healthy subjects. *American Journal of Clinical Nutrition, 72(5)*. 1128-1134.
http://tinyurl.com/HFCS12

Bray, G., et al. (2004, April). Consumption of high fructose corn syrup in beverages may play a role in the epidemic of obesity. *American Journal of Clinical Nutrition, 79(4)*. 537-543.
http://tinyurl.com/HFCS13

Bray, G., et al. (2004, October). Letter to the editor: Reply to MF Jacobson. *American Journal of Clinical Nutrition, 80(4)*. 1081-1082.
http://tinyurl.com/HFCS14

Elliott, S., et al. (2002). Fructose, weight gain, and the insulin resistance syndrome. *American Journal of Clinical Nutrition, 76(5)*. 911.
http://tinyurl.com/HFCS15

Sánchez-Lozada, L,, et al. (2008, November). How safe is fructose for persons with or without diabetes? *American Journal of Clinical Nutrition, 88(11)*. 1189-1190.
http://tinyurl.com/HFCS16

Teff, K., et al. (2004). Dietary fructose reduces circulating insulin and leptin, attenuates postprandial suppression of ghrelin, and increases triglycerides in women. *The Journal of Clinical Endocrinology & Metabolism, 89(6)*. 2963-2972. **http://tinyurl.com/HFCS17**

Richard J. Johnson, MD wrote a book in 2008 about the effects of high-fructose, called "The Sugar Fix". Janice Lorigan wrote one in 2007 entitled "High Fructose Corn Syrup and the Fibromyalgia Connection: Fibromyalgia Recovery Handbook". Nancy Irven and Paulette Lash Ritchie wrote "Please Don't Eat the Wallpaper!: The Teenager's Guide to Avoiding Trans Fats, Enriched Wheat and High

Fructose Corn Syrup" in 2008. I commend all of these authors for recognizing the need for these books.

Documentaries that highlight HFCS include King Corn and Food, Inc.

List of foods containing HFCS: **http://tinyurl.com/HFCSFoods**

List of HFCS-Free Foods: **http://tinyurl.com/HFCSNO**

MSG

Soup manufacturers have begun television advertisements, too. These are not aimed at convincing the consumer that MSG is safe in their products, but rather to publicize that they either already have or plan to remove MSG from their products. And if you see commercials promoting the "umami" taste, that just happens to be the taste of MSG. **http://tinyurl.com/MSGeverywhere**

You might be wondering why anyone would be concerned about MSG, unless they happen to be one of those people that reacts to MSG with a headache, commonly experienced after Chinese food consumption, if it contains MSG. "I'm not one of those people," you might say, "Why would I care if my food has MSG?" Well, let's see, do you have any concerns about becoming obese, depressed, or developing Alzheimer's? Do you care about your children being autistic or having ADHD?

MSG and Obesity

This recent study at University of North Carolina at Chapel Hill published by Johns Hopkins **http://tinyurl.com/MSGstudy** just illustrated some of the things that I said over two years ago.

Do you know how researchers create obese rats and mice for experiments? Well, it is pretty easy to do: you just use MSG. Here are some research studies to show how common this knowledge is among scientists: **http://tinyurl.com/MSGstudy2**

The monosodium glutamate (MSG) obese rat as a model for the study of exercise in obesity. Gobatto CA, Mello MA, Souza CT, Ribeiro IA. Res Commun Mol Pathol Pharmacol. 2002.

Adrenalectomy abolishes the food-induced hypothalamic serotonin release in both normal and monosodium glutamate-obese rats. Guimaraes RB, Telles MM, Coelho VB, Mori RC, Nascimento CM, Ribeiro Brain Res Bull. August 2002.

Obesity induced by neonatal monosodium glutamate treatment in spontaneously hypertensive rats: an animal model of multiple risk factors. Yamamoto M, Iino K, Ichikawa K, Shinohara N, Yoshinari Fujishima Hypertens Res. March 1998.

Hypothalamic lesion induced by injection of monosodium glutamate in suckling period and subsequent development of obesity. Tanaka K, Shimada M, Nakao K, Kusunoki Exp Neurol. October 1978.

Did you notice that the hypothalamic lesions were induced by MSG? Dr. Simeons' theory that damage to the hypothalamus is what causes obesity is alive and well! And we know how to repair that damage, by tricking our bodies into thinking that they are pregnant.

Take a look at all of this research showing that brain and nerve damage is repaired with different pregnancy hormones:

September 2007: One Doctor's Lonely Quest To Heal Brain Injury: After 40 Years, Skeptics Back Hormone Therapy. **http://tinyurl.com/healing1**

May 2007: Pregnancy hormone may help with brain injury. **http://tinyurl.com/healing2**

February 2007: Pregnancy hormone may offer hope for MS patients. Mice study shows how prolactin can repair nerve cells damaged by the disease. **http://tinyurl.com/healing3**

December 2006: Autism Cure? Pregnancy Hormone Offers New Hope. **http://tinyurl.com/healing4**

January 2003: Pregnancy hormone triggers growth of brain cells. **http://tinyurl.com/healing5**

October 2002: Pregnancy hormone estriol Reduces MS Lesions in Small Study. **http://tinyurl.com/healing6**

September 2002: A hormone common in pregnant women shows promise as an easily administered treatment for people with early-stage multiple sclerosis (MS). A new study by UCLA neuroscientists shows for the first time in humans that estriol in oral tablet form can decrease the size and number of brain lesions. **http://tinyurl.com/healing7**

I can hear you now. "But I am very careful to avoid MSG. I look for it on labels before I buy packaged food. I look for 'No MSG' on the label and buy only those foods." That's what I said.

The bad news is that we were both wrong. Despite our good intentions, the food manufacturers were and are one step ahead of us. Remember: By FDA definition, all MSG is "naturally occurring." "Natural" doesn't mean "safe." "Natural" only means that the ingredient started out in nature.

First of all, the label might not state monosodium glutamate or MSG, but the food product could have MSG anyway. How can this be? The FDA, in their infinite wisdom, allows free glutamate to be included in a product and be labeled as an ingredient other than MSG: **http://tinyurl.com/hiddenMSG**

When reading labels, look for the new cloak for MSG, "Natural Flavors". Believe it or not, a company can legally say "There is no MSG in our product" as long as the MSG is a CONSTITUENT of an INGREDIENT such as the ingredient "Natural Flavors". This is extremely deceptive on the part of the government to allow this. I ask, if MSG truly isn't harmful, why is it hidden this way?

Processed Chinese food is higher in MSG than American processed food. The following BBC article states that between 1985 and 2000, overweight and obesity in China's children has increased an extremely alarming *28 fold*. **http://tinyurl.com/MSGChina http://tinyurl.com/MSGFDA**

You might find two studies published in 2005 particularly interesting in light of how much they sound like the mice and rat studies: **http://tinyurl.com/MSGAppetite** and **http://tinyurl.com/MSGAppetite2**

Dr. Russell Blaylock exposed this problem in one of his books: **http://tinyurl.com/MSGBlaylock**

He explains that a neuroscientist Dr. John Olney found out in 1969 that baby rats became morbidly obese when they were fed MSG, an easily repeatable experiment. This connection was first discovered in 1840 when tumors were found in that region of the brain during an autopsy of a woman who had developed an uncontrollable appetite and obesity. Most scientists have known for over five decades that damage, tumors, lesions, or injury to the ventromedial hypothalamus (VMH) would cause obesity and preferential fat storage, even in the absence of excess calories and even in the face of starvation. This is precisely the area of the hypothalamus that is damaged by MSG.

To understand one way that MSG could cause obesity, let's look at an enzyme called AMPK, a protein kinase released in the body during times of stress, in order to limit its use of energy as much as possible, in order to prevent cells from running out of energy and dying. MSG activates AMPK because it is an excitotoxin that causes the cells to use too much energy, in turn triggering the defense of attempting to prevent the loss of more energy.

I'll give you one guess which vulnerable part of the brain is involved with this AMPK enzyme? You don't have to be a rocket scientist to guess that it might be the hypothalamus. In that part of the brain, leptin is an inhibitor of AMPK. MSG-treated mice became leptin-resistant, and with leptin being an AMPK suppressor and MSG being an AMPK activator, MSG could prevent leptin from working as it is intended to do. Interestingly enough, stroke victims also are being treated with glutamate blockers because it is glutamate that causes the stroke damage. The ischemia caused by stroke also causes energy depletion, which in turn causes AMPK to be released as a protective measure. CoQ10 can help to diminish an MSG reaction because as an antioxidant, CoQ10 can help the body to withstand the stress that glutamate induces on the body. If the food industry is not held accountable for its part in the continuing obesity epidemic, there is no justice in the world.

Alzheimer's and MSG

Michael Hermanussen, M.D., a pediatrician in Germany, says the naturally occurring amounts of glutamate aren't the problem; it's the glutamates that the food industry adds to what we eat and drink. Hermanussen has been conducting a study using Memantine, a drug usually used to treat Alzheimer's disease, for weight control, and all of his subjects, he says, have lost weight easily.

Memantine is a member of the class of drugs called glutamate blockers, which keep MSG from reaching glutamate receptors in the brain. More about Memantine: **http://tinyurl.com/Memantine**

Ajinomoto Company, Inc, is the inventor of, and the world's leading producer of, monosodium glutamate; producer of additional MSG-containing ingredients; and the owner and manufacturer of aspartame, another excitotoxin, as described in a review of Dr Blaylock's book, Excitotoxins: The Taste That Kills. **http://tinyurl.com/MSGBlaylock2**

And so here's some research for all of you Conspiracy Theorists.
According to an article in the St. Petersburg Times from September 25, 2005, the drug Memantine is produced by the very same company as the one that manufactures MSG. According to the article, Ajinomoto's pharmaceutical arm, Ajinomoto Pharma, partners with a company called Daiichi Pharmaceuticals. Daiichi partners with Merz Pharmaceuticals. And Merz produces Memantine. That's right. Ajinomoto has a financial interest in Memantine (Namenda), the first drug developed for people with advanced Alzheimer's – a drug that according to the AARP (AARP Bulletin / July-August 2004, p 13), "...blunts the brain chemical glutamate [glutamic acid] which can accumulate abnormally and kill brain cells." Talk about creating your own market...!!!

144

Depression and MSG

Glutamate blockers such as Memantine can also treat long-term, drug-resistant depression. 250,000 people commit suicide in China each year. It is becoming a public health crisis in China.
http://tinyurl.com/ChinaDep
http://tinyurl.com/ChinaDep2

Autism, ADD, ADHD, and MSG

http://tinyurl.com/MSGADHD

How can I avoid MSG if there are so many different names for it?

Good question. It isn't easy. You have to be on the lookout for many many names. For the most part, I would avoid the following ingredients as much as humanly possible: Autolyzed yeast, Calcium caseinate, Glutamate, Glutamic acid, Gelatin, Hydrolyzed corn gluten, Hydrolyzed protein (any protein that is hydrolyzed), Monopotassium glutamate, Monosodium glutamate, MSG, Natrium glutamate (natrium is Latin for sodium), Sodium caseinate, Textured protein, Yeast extract, Yeast food, and Yeast nutrient. Also, if you are in Europe, MSG is referred to on labels as E621 and it's not very intuitive to figure out that E621 means MSG, is it?

And then we have the processed food ingredients that quite often will create MSG while being prepared: Anything enzyme modified, Anything fermented, Anything protein fortified, Barley malt, Bouillon and Broth, Carrageenan, Citric acid, Enzymes anything, Flavors(s) and Flavoring(s), Malt extract, Malt flavoring, Maltodextrin, Natural beef flavoring, Natural chicken flavoring, Natural flavor(s) and flavoring(s), Natural pork flavoring, Pectin, Protease, Protease enzymes, Seasonings (the actual word "seasonings"), Soy protein, Soy protein concentrate, Soy protein isolate, Soy sauce, Soy sauce extract, Stock, Ultra-pasteurized, Whey protein, Whey protein concentrate, and Whey protein isolate. You can see why I prefer egg protein over the soy and the whey, now.

More tricks used to hide MSG

The Dead Give Away... If you see either disodium guanylate or disodium inosinate in a list of ingredients, the product probably also contains MSG. These are expensive food additives that work synergistically with inexpensive MSG. Their use suggests that the product has MSG in it. They would probably not be used as food additives if there were no MSG present.

MSG in products other than processed foods

MSG reactions have been reported to soaps, shampoos, hair conditioners, and cosmetics, where MSG is hidden in ingredients that include the words "hydrolyzed," "amino acids," and "protein."

Low fat and no fat dairy products often include milk solids that contain MSG, which is yet another reason to avoid those fake foods.

Drinks, candy, and chewing gum are potential sources of hidden MSG and of aspartame and neotame. Aspartic acid, found in neotame and aspartame (NutraSweet), ordinarily causes MSG type reactions in MSG sensitive people. Aspartame is found in some medications, including children's medications. Neotame is relatively new and I have not yet seen it used widely.

Binders and fillers for medications, nutrients, and supplements, both prescription and non-prescription, enteral feeding materials, and some fluids administered intravenously in hospitals, may contain MSG.

According to the manufacturer, Varivax–Merck chicken pox vaccine (Varicella Virus Live), contains L-monosodium glutamate and hydrolyzed gelatin, both of which contain processed free glutamic acid (MSG) It would appear that most, if not all, live virus vaccines contain MSG.

And the topper: Folks, they are even spraying our crops with MSG, if you can believe that. AuxiGro® is MSG sprayed on crops to make them grow. On January 14, 1998, AuxiGro®, which contains processed free glutamic acid, was registered as a growth enhancer with the EPA (U.S. Environmental Protection Agency). Permission was given to spray it on all agricultural products. Plants sprayed with AuxiGro® receive a false signal that they are under "stress" and respond by pulling more nutrients from the soil and thus grow much larger, increasing yields. The recent huge potatoes and yams in the supermarket appear to be a direct result of AuxiGro®.

So How Should I Eat to Maintain?

Dr Simeons stated flat out that he only had a 70% long-term success rate. If you don't want to be part of the 30% that relapsed into obesity again, I believe that you must abandon most what you've been taught about nutrition and health for the past 30 years. Approach Phase 4, the rest of your life, as a great adventure in finding out just what you can eat and maintain, and in finding out how your appetite and food preferences have changed. Eating 40% fat, 30-40% protein, and 20-30% carbohydrates in my diet most days works for me. That is not to say that I don't eat more carbs on some days, but the day after, I return to those percentages. I thought about recommending that for everyone, but if there is one thing that I have learned in my support group, it is that we are all different. What I am reasonably sure about is what the optimum nutrition and healthy diet for you will NOT be:
- It will not be based upon avoiding cholesterol or eating low-fat or non-fat foods. None other than Dr Michael DeBakey said that in thousands, he had seen no significant, consistent correlation between cholesterol levels and arteriosclerosis. **http://tinyurl.com/DeBakey http://tinyurl.com/DeBakey2**
- It will not be based upon eating 6 to 11 servings of grains per day, and correspondingly less fat, which was a government experiment (the food pyramid) gone horribly wrong. Harvard School of Public Health reported that when we were eating 45% fat, 13% were obese and less than 1% had diabetes. Reducing the fat to 33% resulted in 34% obesity rates and 8% diabetes incidence. Do you think that's a coincidence? I don't. **http://tinyurl.com/PerCentFat**

Final Tribute to Dr. Simeons

I would like to conclude this book with a commemorative link to a photo of Dr Alfred Theodore William Simeons' gravestone at Acattolico Cemetery (the old cemetery for non-Catholic foreigners) in Rome: **http://tinyurl.com/SimeonsGrave** When you see what this diet does for you, Dr Simeons will mean something very special and precious to you as he does to me.

hCG Checklist

This plan works much better if you plan and prepare. This is a list that I used to ensure that I did not forget anything. You may print this list out and check off the items with a pen.

☐ 1. Read this book in its entirety.
☐ 2. Take a "before" picture of yourself. Yes, it is humbling, but you will be glad you did later, when it is time for a side by side comparison of before and after.
☐ 3. Take your "before" measurements. Again, you will be happy that you did.
☐ 4. Read Dr. Simeons' "Pounds and Inches".
☐ 5. Apply to join the HCG Diet Made Simple support group by sending an email to: HCGDietMadeSimple-subscribe@yahoogroups.com.
☐ 6. Take stock of your personal readiness state. Answer the following questions for yourself:
☐   o Can you commit to staying on the program for the time needed?
☐   o How easily can you fit the program into your lifestyle?
☐   o What opposition will you have from family and friends?
☐   o What support will you have from family and friends?
☐   o Will you have the support and help of your doctor?
☐   o Will you be confident enough to do the program on your own, or do you need to use a clinic to provide you with meds and support?
☐   o Do you have the financial means to purchase the needed supplies?
☐   o Do you have the time needed to complete at least one round?
☐   o Are you ready to change your life?
☐ 7. Decide if you need a new scale to weigh your body.
☐ 8. Read "Pounds and Inches" AGAIN!!!
☐ 9. Approach your doctor about the protocol, if you choose to do so.
☐ 10. Determine whether your doctor will be supportive or actually prescribe the hCG for you.
☐ 11. If your doctor will not support you, review the Clinics section of the book.
☐ 12. Decide whether to use a clinic or go it on your own.
☐ 13. Choose a clinic, if needed.
☐ 14. If doing this without a clinic or physician:
☐   o Decide whether to do Subcutaneous or Intramuscular injections OR use a sublingual mixture.
☐   o Determine how much hCG you will need to lose the weight you want.
☐   5. What dosage will you take?
☐   6. How many rounds do you need to do?
☐   7. Will other family or friends be doing the program with you?
☐   o Review the hCG suppliers section of the book and decide where to order hCG.
☐   o Order hCG.
☐   o Review the book sections for your chosen administration method and determine what supplies for giving injections or mixing sublingual that you need to purchase.
☐   o Order supplies.
☐ 15. Plan your program by deciding your schedule for Phases and rounds, considering holidays, vacations, and special events.
☐ 16. If necessary, buy scales for weighing yourself and your food.
☐ 17. Become educated about Cleanses for Phase 1.
☐ 18. Purchase and use cleanses and other Phase I options, if you choose to do so.
☐ 19. Become educated about organic food.
☐ 20. Determine sources for organic food, if you choose to do so.
☐ 21. Begin purchasing and eating organic, if you choose to do so.

- [ ] 22. Visit **www.hcgdietingstore.com** to see some products that can be used on the protocol.
- [ ] 23. Change to protocol-compliant personal care products, if you choose to do so.
- [ ] 24. Mentally prepare for Phase 2.
- [ ] 25. Review the section in the book on the Recipes for the diet plan and food preparation.
- [ ] 26. Plan your Phase 2 meals for the first week using the Meal Planning Auto Calorie Calculator Spreadsheet.
- [ ] 27. Set interim goals for yourself so that you can celebrate your success along the way.
- [ ] 28. If doing this on your own, on the first day of Phase 2, mix the hCG and store it properly.
- [ ] 29. Begin your hCG administration method of choice.
- [ ] 30. Decide how to handle other people while on the diet.
- [ ] 31. Weigh yourself each day and record the weight in the Pounds and Inches Tracking Spreadsheet.
- [ ] 32. Load TO CAPACITY with lots of fats for the first two days of hCG administration.
- [ ] 33. Begin the 500 calorie food plan (VLCD) on day three.
- [ ] 34. Record your food each day, to be used for analysis purposes later, if not reducing weight.
- [ ] 35. If continuing Phase 2 past 23 days, skip hCG one day a week, but continue 500 calories on that day.
- [ ] 36. If you remain at the same weight for four days, you may do an apple day, as described on pages 68-69 of "Pounds and Inches".
- [ ] 37. Begin your preparation mentally for Phase 3.
- [ ] 38. One week before discontinuation of hCG, begin planning Phase 3 meals with no refined sugar or starch. Do NOT limit fat, salt, or anything else. Plan in particular for much more protein, as you are on the verge of protein deficiency when beginning Phase 3.
- [ ] 39. Review the Phase 3 lists of sugars and starches.
- [ ] 40. Record your weight on your last injection or sublingual dose day. This is your LIW.
- [ ] 41. Continue 500 calories for 72 hours after the last injection. You may continue to lose on these days.
- [ ] 42. Review the sample Phase 3 menu. Do NOT continue 500 calories after this. It is very important to eat MUCH more food and in particular, protein, for three weeks. Eat foods that were not allowed in Phase 2, but still do not have refined sugar or starch. Do NOT be afraid of fat. Use full-fat products, NOT low-fat or non-fat.
- [ ] 43. Continue to weigh yourself daily in Phase 3.
- [ ] 44. If you weigh more than 2 pounds over your last injection weight or last sublingual dose weight on any day, you must do a steak day on that day as described on pages 92-93 of "Pounds and Inches". Do not wait. Do it that day.
- [ ] 45. If you suspect that you have edema (water retention) caused by insufficient protein, do the eggs-steak-cheese day as described on page 96 of "Pounds and Inches".
- [ ] 46. After completing three weeks of no refined sugar or starches, you may proceed to Phase 4, gradually adding sugars and starches. Dr. Simeons requires three weeks of Phase 4 before beginning your second round of Phase 2, If needed. If you have reached your goal weight, CELEBRATE!!!

Calorie Calculator and Food Record

Day/Date			
Food Item	Ca/Oz	Oz eaten	Calories
Apple, raw	15		
Grapefruit, raw	9		
Orange, raw	13		
Strawberries, raw	9		
Asparagus, raw	6		
Beet Greens	6		
Cabbage	7		
Celery	4		
Chard	7		
Chicory	7		
Cucumber	3		
Fennel	9		
Lettuce,Romaine	5		
Lettuce, Iceburg	4		
Onion, bulb raw	12		
Onion, green	9		
Radish	5		
Spinach	7		
Tomatoes, raw	5		
Chicken, raw	31		
Crawfish	27		
Flounder/Sole	26		
Halibut	31		
Hamburger 85% lean	60		
Hamburger 90% Lean	50		
Hamburger 95% Lean	38		
Prawn	30		
Steak, sirloin	37		
Scallops	25		
Shrimp, shelled	30		
Lemon Juice-Wedge	1		
DAILY CALORIE TOTAL			
CALORIES LEFT			
Tea			
Water			

Pounds and Inches Tracking Chart

Date	Weight (lbs.)	Pounds change	Chest (in.)	Waist (in.)	Tummy (in.)	Hips (in.)	Thigh L (in.)	Thigh R (in.)	Arm L	Arm R	Total inches

COUPON

FREE coupon for a 5-minute phone consultation with Victoria Smith, Candida and Detox Expert ($30 value) after you fill out this coupon and email to: victoria@significanthealing.com.

Name: _____

Address: _____

Required: Book order transaction number: _____

LaVergne, TN USA
26 July 2010
190951LV00006BA/55/P